The Complete Idiot's Reference Card

tear here

How to Eat

1. Reduce stress before eating.
2. Eat beautifully in a relaxing environment.
3. Eat slowly, taking at least 15 to 20 minutes per meal.
4. Eat while sitting down.
5. Eat about as much food as the size of your fist.

Hunger Scale

Tune into your stomach's hunger feelings:

(0)	(5)	(7)	(10)
empty	satisfied	full	stuffed
hungry	comfortable	ate too much	
time to eat	time to stop		

Rules for using the hunger scale:

1. Eat only when your stomach registers zero (0).
2. Eat enough to be satisfied or comfortable, that is, up to five (5).
3. Stop eating before you are full (7).
4. If you should overeat, that is, eat above five (5), forgive yourself and wait until you are at zero (0) before you eat again.

How to Eat Balanced Proteins, Carbs, and Fats

At every meal and snack, eat foods in the following approximate ratios:

High-quality protein	35 to 50 percent
Low- to moderate-glycemic carbs	30 to 50 percent
Fats	20 to 30 percent

Use Your Mental Power

1. Use affirmations, visualizations, and intentions daily.
2. Write forgivenesses as a way to release past emotions.
3. Get rid of anything in your home that a thin person wouldn't own.
4. Clean out anything in your home or life that is stuffed: drawers, garage, handbag, and your to-do list.
5. Pretend you already are at your ideal size.

ALPHA

Avoid Starvation Metabolism

1. Eat only when you are hungry.
2. Don't skip meals when you are hungry.
3. Eat a balanced diet that includes protein, carbohydrates, and fat.
4. Avoid extreme diets and starvation diets.
5. Never overeat if you've let yourself get too hungry.
6. Consume a daily dose of essential fatty acids and high-quality protein.
7. Don't even think that starving yourself or missing meals is the way to lose weight.

Boost Your Metabolism

1. Eat 0 to 5 on the hunger scale.
2. Increase muscle mass and decrease body fat percentage through exercise.
3. Get adequate sleep every night.
4. Drink eight 8-ounce glasses (or more) of water per day.
5. Reduce chronic stress.
6. Avoid eating artificial foods.
7. Eat low- to moderate-glycemic carbohydrates and avoid eating high-glycemic carbohydrates.
8. Stay out of starvation metabolism.
9. Exercise three to seven times a week.
10. Don't eat foods you are allergic to.

Exercise Guidelines

1. Set up an exercise plan that includes these three components:

    Cardio—a minimum of 20 minutes at least three times a week. More is great!

    Strength training—do two to three sessions a week.

    Flexibility—stretch before and after workouts and/or do one to two stretching sessions per week.
2. Increase intensity as your body adapts to new levels of fitness.
3. Schedule exercise appointments in your daily planner and keep your appointments.
4. Enjoy recreational exercise through activities such as dancing, hiking, tennis, and swimming.
5. Value exercise and enjoy it—it helps get you to and keep you at your ideal size.

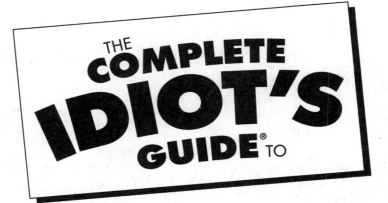

THE COMPLETE IDIOT'S GUIDE® TO

Weight Loss

by Lucy Beale
and
Sandy G. Couvillon, MS, LDN, RD
with
Katherine A. Hutcheson, Ed.D. and
Beverly Donnelley, MD

ALPHA

A Pearson Education Company

13671599

Lucy: To Patrick
Sandy: To my Mom and Dad

Copyright © 2003 by Lucy Beale and Sandy G. Couvillon

International Standard Book Number: 0-02864385-2
Library of Congress Catalog Card Number: 2002111652

04   03   02   8   7   6   5   4   3   2   1

Interpretation of the printing code: The rightmost number of the first series of numbers is the year of the book's printing; the rightmost number of the second series of numbers is the number of the book's printing. For example, a printing code of 02-1 shows that the first printing occurred in 2002.

Printed in the United States of America

For marketing and publicity, please call: 317-581-3722

The publisher offers discounts on this book when ordered in quantity for bulk purchases and special sales.

For sales within the United States, please contact: Corporate and Government Sales, 1-800-382-3419 or corpsales@pearsontechgroup.com.

Outside the United States, please contact: International Sales, 317-581-3793 or international@pearsontechgroup.com.

Publisher: *Marie Butler-Knight*
Product Manager: *Phil Kitchel*
Managing Editor: *Jennifer Chisholm*
Acquisitions Editor: *Mike Sanders*
Development Editor: *Nancy D. Lewis*
Production Editor: *Katherin Bidwell*
Copy Editor: *Amy Lepore*
Illustrator: *Chris Eliopoulos*
Cover/Book Designer: *Trina Wurst*
Indexer: *Angie Bess*
Layout/Proofreading: *Megan Douglass, Brad Lenser*

Contents at a Glance

Contents

Foreword

I love this book and you will, too! Lucy Beale's work is the epitome of leading-edge thinking when it comes to reshaping the body and the mind. Lucy and her co-author, Sandy Couvillon, reveal the ultimate principles to change your lifestyle and live in your ideal, healthy, and fit body!

I met Lucy Beale in 1998 when I was well over the 300-pound mark. When I say well over, I mean my midriff drifted around my body, covering my hips and resting on my thighs when I sat down. I was not a pretty picture. And I was miserable. I had no self-esteem, hated the body I lived in, and was terribly depressed. Fortunately, somewhere in my brain there was still a cell that believed I could overcome obesity, and that cell somehow found Lucy Beale … just like you have found this book.

Lucy taught me to stop telling myself I was fat when I awoke every morning, to start being kind to myself, and, most importantly, to begin communicating immediately with my body. I had never heard of the 0-to-5 hunger scale, and this ingenious strategy taught me to get in touch with my body. After a few months of using Lucy's philosophy, I called her up and told her, "Lucy, I have never really lived in my body!"

When I was overweight, I always felt empty and kept feeding the feeling. That feeling of emptiness was my body and mind trying to get my attention! My body was not empty … it just wasn't fulfilled. In changing my attitudes and behaviors toward food, eating, and my body, I became aware of my body's intelligence. I learned that my body was a great communicator. It always tells me exactly what it wants. My job is to listen and respond responsibly.

The exercise suggestions in the book include some simple ones that have become for me a precious daily gift to my body. Just 10 minutes a day have been enough to help me reach my ideal size and rid myself of a yucky double chin.

Today, several years after adopting Lucys system, I am five clothing sizes smaller and happier than ever. I used to wear a size 26. Now I wear a size 16. Keeping weight off is no longer the struggle it was in the past.

By following the life-changing principles in this book, you will create a loving relationship with your body. You will want to feed your body just the right amount of wonderful, healthy foods, to take your body for a walk or to a yoga class, and to clothe it in something that reveals its shape! Lucy and Sandy's approach does take some effort, but nothing compared to the struggle of living life as an overweight person. Getting to your ideal size is a life-changing transformation that will make you feel fulfilled, improve your self-esteem, and give you the healthy life you have always desired.

Take this book and devour it! It will be the first time in your life you overindulge something that will make you naturally thin! I know. I have lived the principles in this book and my reflection in the mirror is one I love!

—Deborah Miles Kelly

Introduction

Yes, you can get to an ideal size that is realistic for you and stay there for life. You can master your eating and your weight. In this book, you will learn how and what to eat, how to think, how to exercise, and how to avoid common weight-loss pitfalls. We won't teach you some gimmicky solution. Instead, you learn the basics that help you lose weight faster and stay healthier. Simple, smart, common-sense approaches are the hallmark of this book.

Start now to plan your new thinner wardrobe and attitude. You can have the results you want and deserve.

How This Book Is Organized

The book is divided into six parts:

Part 1, "What Size Do You Want to Be?" guides you to determine the body size that's best for you. You'll learn about being overweight, the obesity epidemic, and the health risks of excessive weight. Just as important, we'll dispel popular weight myths and replace them with confidence-boosting knowledge, practical advice, and inspiration to get you started on the right path, right away.

Part 2, "Your Body of Information," introduces you to how your body handles food and eating and what causes it to either gain or lose weight. You will learn to appreciate your body and its appetite, to boost your body's natural metabolic rate, and to avoid self-defeating starvation metabolism. You'll master simple ways to make eating a relaxed, beautiful part of your life and to soothe stress and avoid anxiety in eating situations.

Part 3, "Using Food to Support Your Weight Loss," will give you an understanding of what foods you need for healthy weight loss. You'll read a straightforward explanation of the essential qualities of proteins, fats, and carbohydrates and how you should balance them in your safe, nutritional eating plan. Plus, you'll get valuable insight into using nutritional supplements.

Part 4, "Exercise Is Your Friend," explores why exercise is an essential part of developing a healthy body that provides you with a nice body shape, muscle tone, and stamina. We debunk exercise myths and fads and show you how to put together a home program that will help you look good and feel good. You also learn how to incorporate recreational exercise into your lifestyle.

Part 5, "Understanding Weight-Loss Plans," analyzes popular weight-loss plans to steer you to the ones that will work best for you. You'll have a chance to see which ones are gimmicky (maybe even unsafe) and which ones are based on sound principles. We also discuss fad diets and medical approaches.

Part 6, "Get Your Mindset Right," uses the principles of the body-mind connection to teach you how visualizations and affirmations can hasten your weight-loss progress. You will learn how to approach dining out, family holidays, and vacations with confidence and ease, knowing that you can continue your progress at all times.

Extra Bites

The sidebars in this book offer tips, inspiration, valuable knowledge, and definitions. Use these as road signs on the journey to your goal—your ideal size.

Lean Lingo
The definitions of words and concepts in these boxes will expand your knowledge of weight loss, nutrition, and health terms ... without expanding your waist.

Thinspiration
Like a friendly weight-loss coach, these boxes contain positive, inspiring, and uplifting thoughts plus encouragement for your journey from over-weight to thin.

Weighty Warning
Mistakes happen, but these warnings should help keep you from stalling your progress and making fattening mistakes.

Body of Knowledge
These facts increase your knowledge base for life-long weight maintenance.

Acknowledgments

Our dream of writing a practical and inspiring guide to weight loss couldn't have become a reality without, first and foremost, our clients and students who have egged us on to find solutions to their weight-loss problems. We appreciate each and every one of you.

Lucy Beale would like to give a special thanks to her loving husband, Patrick Partridge, for his late-night manuscript reviews, enthusiasm, and hugs; to Bob DiForio, Marilyn Allen, and Coleen O'Shea for their constant support and belief in a weight-loss book; and to the readers of her *Thinspirations* newsletter who continue to inform and inspire her efforts. A special thank you goes to her son, Brian, who taught her about meaningful learning and love.

Thanks to Connie Mahaffey, Dr. Brian Martin, Dr. Tyteeka Reye, Dr. Steve Nugent, Caryll Cram, Steve Burns, and Lynette Reiling for generously sharing information and support.

Sandy Couvillon gives special thanks to her husband, Brian, for his love and confidence in her. He never once complained as she went through tons of research and sat at the computer for hours. Love and laughter go to her adult children, Courtney and Brad, for years of sampling unfamiliar foods for their "dietitian mom." Much love to her parents, Jim and Velma Guess, who have always believed that she knew her stuff. Sandy appreciates her family for supporting her utmost career desire to educate and impact others with compassion and wisdom. She loves you all dearly.

Our many thanks to Mike Sanders and the editorial team at Alpha who made this book a reality. Finally, we would like to thank you, our reader, because you have acquired this book to help you master your weight. Many of you are frustrated and seeking sound guidance, and we are pleased you have chosen this roadmap on your journey to reach your ideal size. Please let us know when you get there!

Trademarks

All terms mentioned in this book that are known to be or are suspected of being trademarks or service marks have been appropriately capitalized. Alpha Books and Pearson Education, Inc., cannot attest to the accuracy of this information. Use of a term in this book should not be regarded as affecting the validity of any trademark or service mark.

Part 1

What Size Do You Want to Be?

If reaching your ideal size and staying there were as simple as popping a pill, you wouldn't be reading this book. Nor would we have today's obesity epidemic in the United States. As a nation, we're getting "larger" every year, despite all the low-fat foods, crash diets, and eating systems we're being asked to buy into.

This part of the book starts you on your journey toward your ideal body by teaching you some fundamental guiding principles. You'll learn about health risks associated with being overweight and some very real benefits of maintaining a healthy weight. You'll learn some of the real causes of being overweight (and the myths), how to intelligently choose your ideal size, and some attitude adjustments that will help you succeed. You'll gather in up-to-date knowledge, practical advice, and simple inspirations that will make you realize "I can do it!" In fact, we're confident you *will* do it.

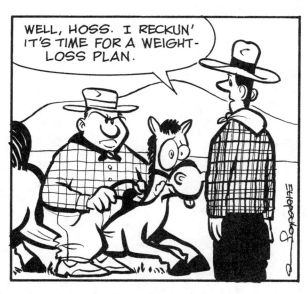

Chapter 1

The Joy of Being Your Ideal Size

In This Chapter

- The U.S. obesity epidemic
- Health risks of being overweight or obese
- Preparation for weight loss
- Very real benefits of living at your ideal size

Picture yourself the way you want to look. That's the image to hold in your head as you read this book. It's also the self-image you should keep for the rest of your life—because that's the way you *can* look!

For now, however, you've got a weight issue. Perhaps you're carrying 15 pounds and a few more inches than your ideal. Maybe it's 50 pounds or more. Perhaps you've tried different diets and food plans, along with various exercise regimes. Most likely, your long-term results have been disappointing. While you may have lost weight at times, eventually something happened and you regained the weight, perhaps even more than you lost. Worse, you are at a loss to know why your best efforts have failed.

You know there must be a solution to your weight issue. After all, aren't there plenty of people who both enjoy food and stay at their ideal size, the size that is realistic for them? The good news is that you can be one of them! That's the fundamental message of this book.

A Nation Getting Fatter

You are not alone. The U.S. population is larger than ever before in history. Gradually we have become a land of "supersized" individuals. Over 65 percent of American adults are *overweight* or obese today. That means over 97.1 million adults in the United States are unsuccessful at managing their weight.

> **Lean Lingo** _____
>
> The medical definition of **overweight** is having a body mass index (BMI) of between 25 and 29.9. If your BMI is between 18.5 and 24.9, you are within the normal weight range. If your BMI is higher than 29.9, you are considered to be obese. To calculate your BMI, multiply your weight in pounds by 704.5, divide the result by your height in inches, and then divide that result by your height in inches a second time. See Chapter 3 for more information on BMI.

The U.S. population has been getting progressively weightier for the past four decades. The overweight and obese population has increased from 24.4 percent in 1960 to 65 percent in 2001.

Here's how it breaks down:

    24.4% in 1960-62

    24.9% in 1971-74

    25.4% in 1976-80

    34.8% in 1988-94

    65% in 2001

The trend is not slowing. More and more people are getting bigger. The Centers for Disease Control considers obesity to be a frightening medical epidemic. In 2000, a total of 97.1 million U.S. adults met the criteria for being overweight, and 39.8 million U.S. adults met the criteria for obesity. About 19.6 million men and 19.2 million women are obese. That's a 61 percent increase since 1991—in just 9 years. In 1991, only 4 of 45 states that participated in a National Institute of Health study had obesity rates of 15 to 19 percent of their adult populations. By 2000, 49 states—Colorado was the one exception—had rates of 15 percent or greater. Twenty-two of the 50 states had obesity rates of 20 percent or higher.

What's causing our collective chubbiness? Various pundits place the blame on our sedentary lifestyle, fast food, convenience foods, and processed foods. There simply isn't one cause, nor is there a magic pill or potion that will shrink the population back to size. Being overweight is a condition of lifestyle and poor eating habits, and it can only change when each individual, like you, makes significant and life-enhancing lifestyle changes.

> **Body of Knowledge**
>
> The body mass index (BMI) is not a perfect guide, but it is a useful one. There are a few obvious exceptions to the formula: Athletes with very high muscle mass will have a higher BMI, and people, such as the elderly, who have lost a great amount of muscle mass due to reduced nutritional reserves will have a low BMI.

You Can Buck the Trend

Does it make you feel better that so many others are fighting fat, too? Of course it does. Misery loves company, but you're reading this book because you don't want to be part of that crowd. Don't let the statistics discourage you. It might seem inevitable that a person wouldn't have a fighting chance to buck the trend. If everyone is getting fatter, why shouldn't you expect to be overweight also? Here's the simple answer: because you can be your *ideal size*.

Here are five critical and inspirational points to remember as you use this book and lose those pounds:

1. **You get to choose.** Plenty of people—at least 35 percent of the U.S. population—are *not* overweight. You can be one of them. You are not destined to be fat. You have a choice.

2. **You can learn.** You can master the tried-and-true basics of what and how to eat and how to live as a *thin* person.

3. **You can change.** Many formerly overweight people are enjoying the newfound freedom of being their *ideal size* and enjoying food. If they can do it, so can you.

> **Lean Lingo**
>
> **Thin** is a loaded word. It means different things to different people. In this book, we use it to describe someone at or near the normal range for BMI. Your **ideal size** is the one that keeps you healthy and makes you happy.

Weighty Warning

Obesity is the cause of death of more than 375,000 U.S. adults each year. A person who is obese or overweight is more likely to develop heart disease, strokes, hypertension, diabetes, and certain cancers, which are leading causes of death.

Body of Knowledge

Only about 15 percent of the female population in the United States are "normal eaters." This refers to women who eat according to hunger without preoccupation with body size or weight.

4. **You have the desire.** You obviously have an interest in losing weight. Now you just need to develop the motivation and the wisdom to avoid the fads and the gimmicks that lead to failure. You have the wherewithal to do what works.

5. **You can count on us as knowledgeable friends.** In this book, we tell you what works and what doesn't. You're holding in your hands a friendly guide to reach your size goal. We won't be preachy. We'll show you which exercise and eating changes to make, how to learn from the inevitable mistakes, and how to stay on track for the long term.

So be confident. The fact that others—many others—are overweight does not predict your fate. Join those who have learned how to eat, what to eat, and how to exercise. Join those who get into their smaller jeans easily. They experience the joy of being free of having a weight problem. So will you.

Your beliefs are a powerful force, so believe you have your ideal body even though you aren't there already. Believe you are already there. If inconsistent thoughts or actions arise, change them. To create your ideal size, you must create your thoughts and actions accordingly.

Losing Weight Just Ain't What It Used to Be

As recently as 20 years ago, the common thinking about weight loss was simply to eat fewer calories and do more exercise to burn off the calories, and you would easily get to your ideal size. Few people were successful with this formula, and few can be successful using it today. What research shows is that calories overall don't count as much as which foods you eat and how you eat them. We now know that certain foods stimulate hormones that direct weight gain and loss. These include insulin and cortisol, which are discussed further in Chapters 8 and 12. We know that certain exercises are more effective than others. We know how metabolism works, and we are learning more every day.

Get to Your Ideal Size and Get Healthier

Here's a simple, sobering health fact: Thin is healthier; fatter is riskier. The serious health risks associated with being overweight are an alarming aspect of the growing "size" of the U.S. population. The old-fashioned image of a "fat and happy" person belies the jeopardy of chronic health conditions from obesity. Many individuals are familiar with the increased risk of type 2 diabetes, but the problem doesn't stop there.

The following are known health risks for obesity and being overweight:

◆ Diabetes (type 2)

◆ Heart disease

◆ Stroke

◆ High blood pressure

◆ Gallbladder disease

◆ Osteoarthritis

◆ Sleep apnea and other breathing problems

◆ Cancer (uterine, breast, colorectal, kidney, gallbladder, endometrial)

◆ Gout

Obesity is also associated with the following:

◆ High cholesterol

◆ Pregnancy complications

◆ Menstrual irregularities

◆ Stress incontinence

◆ Psychological disorders such as depression

◆ Increased risk during surgery

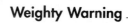

Weighty Warning

Almost half of post-menopausal women diagnosed with breast cancer have a body mass index (BMI) equal to or over 29. The Centers for Disease Control considers a person with a BMI over 29.9 to be obese.

Obese individuals have a 50- to 100-percent increased risk of death from all causes compared with normal-weight individuals. Perhaps you already have some of these health issues. By getting to your ideal size, you are doing one of the best things you can to protect and improve your health. For example, people who are obese have 30 to 50 percent more chronic medical problems than smokers or problem drinkers.

Get to Your Ideal Size and Enjoy How You Look

You want to look your best. You want to fit into your favorite jeans. You want to make an appearance, turn heads, and receive compliments. You want to feel sensuous and desirable when wearing a swimsuit or going to a party or class reunion. Few of us have the genetics to have the figure of a fashion model, but by golly, we want to have shapes we are proud of.

Is this the wrong reason to want to be thinner? Would the world be a better place if we all were less vain? Perhaps. But wanting to look your best is a powerful motivator. Very few people are immune to the urge. You can be sure that no naturally thin person is itching to be overweight!

It isn't fun to feel fat in your clothes. It isn't fun to shop for clothing that hides your size. It isn't fun to be physically uncomfortable in airplane seats. It isn't fun to huff and puff up the steps or to avoid health clubs because you're embarrassed by how you look.

Are you a shallow person just because you want to be at your ideal size to look better? Of course not. Everyone has vanity and glamour needs. (If we didn't, we would all wear the same outfits, no makeup, and the same shoes. How boring!) What would be shallow is to deny the importance you place on how you look. Be honest with yourself.

Note that we aren't talking about becoming "skinny." ("Skinny" is a word that's hard to define, but somehow we all recognize a truly skinny person.) People who starve themselves to the point of frailty to look pencil thin are taking serious health risks.

This book is *not* about attempting to copy the look of the latest *Vogue* models. It's designed to help you reach your *healthy* ideal size.

Life is challenging enough without being self-conscious about your looks. Worrying about your weight is debilitating and doesn't let you shine and radiate happiness. Later on in this book, you will learn to develop the "mindset" of a naturally thin person. But for now, just try to imagine the simple, everyday joy of appreciating your own looks.

Thinspiration

Feeling good about your looks enhances your self-esteem and makes you more courageous, more confident, and more attractive—both to yourself and to others.

Become More Visible

One of our clients, Mary, commented that the biggest difference for her when she went from a size 18 to a size 8 was that she became "visible." Before, Mary could stand and stand at a cosmetic counter in a big department store and never be helped, while those around her were served. Today, the clerks at stores "see" her. They want to sell her cosmetics, clothing, or whatever. At a size 18, Mary was embarrassed to walk into a restaurant. Now when she walks into a restaurant, she is greeted right away and she feels comfortable and welcome.

You can become more visible, too, so get familiar with this concept now and plan to enjoy being visible. Be prepared to accept the responsibility and the resultant delights.

Thinspiration

Right now is a good time to start imagining what it will be like for you to be "visible." Imagine walking into a department store or a restaurant as a trim person. What does it feel like to be noticed? Get ready now, for this will happen as you release body fat. Some people who lose weight find it somewhat scary and intimidating to be "seen." Prepare yourself now. Just for fun, the next time you enter a nice restaurant dressed appropriately, imagine being "visible" like a famous movie star. Make an entrance. Let yourself feel glamorous. If you think it would be too hard to actually do this, let your imagination play out the fantasy.

Look Forward to More Romance

It's probably fortunate that romantic attraction between men and women is more mystery and magic than science. We are attracted to each other for a host of reasons, and physical looks is only one of them. But physical attraction based on looks is certainly very real.

Feeling desirable can have a direct effect on the quality of your romantic life. By contrast, feeling fat can hinder one's love life. Being perceived as fat hinders it even more.

Sadly, this is true even in long-term, loving relationships. Physical attraction can diminish when one or both partners become overweight. We hear it all the time from clients.

Should you be angry about it? No! Go ahead and focus on romance now by making yourself as desirable as possible at your current size. Then proceed to get to your ideal size … and look forward to enjoying extra sizzle in your romantic life.

Body of Knowledge

In the world of online romantic personals, it's said that men lie most about their height and women lie most about their weight. You know the reason. A woman who is overweight feels undesirable. She fears that fewer men want to date and marry overweight women. Men generally want to be taller as this is associated with power and virility.

Get to Your Ideal Size and Join in on Financial Rewards

Get rid of the excess inches by depositing them in the bank! Okay, you can't literally do that, but there are often professional and income benefits from reaching your ideal size. Over time, the extra income can add considerably to your bank account.

Workplace discrimination against overweight people is seldom discussed and certainly not openly acknowledged, but you know it's there. You feel it. You may have been told in some ambiguous way that, if you don't lose weight, you will be passed over for promotion or, even worse, will be downsized. ("Downsized" is not a happy word in this context.) Perhaps you have already been derailed or knocked out of the running for a promotion and pay increase while a less-qualified-but-thin colleague got the job you deserved. You may never be able to prove you were discriminated against, but you know.

Yes, this is illegal, and it's infuriating. In its most blatant forms, it's obnoxious and even immoral. But that doesn't make it less real. Many of our clients have recounted sad stories of such job discrimination. We can only hope that weight discrimination will decrease over time, but don't count on it happening soon.

The real problem may be much more subtle. Those who discriminate may be doing so entirely subconsciously. Research by John Cawley of the University of Michigan has shown that a white woman who is perceived as being overweight may earn 7 percent less in pay than a woman who is perceived to be at her ideal size. In a 40-year work career with an estimated annual salary of $30,000, the average overweight woman can lose $84,000 in earning power. Think about how many vacations and pairs of shoes that money could buy!

If you are in a profession in which you have direct contact with customers and the public, your perceived size can make a big difference in your performance and pay. Why? Because you are subjected to people's underlying prejudices about those who are overweight—even if they are overweight themselves. Many professional salespersons, especially women, who are at their ideal size earn more than those who are overweight.

> ### Body of Knowledge
> Both men and women who are overweight may be discriminated against, but men typically have more "room" to be a bit portly before size discrimination sets in.

Plenty of individuals who are themselves overweight are hypercritical of other overweight individuals. Go figure. They seem to recognize their own issues and project them onto others who live in overweight bodies. It doesn't make much sense and isn't pretty, but it is a fact.

What is a person to do? Get to your ideal size and stay there. If you're a woman, you may be giving yourself a 7-percent raise. The best and easiest way to deal with these unfortunate facts is to work with them. By the way, this doesn't mean you need to accept the prejudice or the implicit underlying assumptions that prejudiced people make. The assumptions aren't kind, noble, or loving, but we all have irrational prejudices. Get to your ideal size for personal reasons and, in the process, attain your professional and personal goals and ensuing rewards. Then, when you're in a position of authority, make sure you never, never discriminate against someone with a weight issue … because you've been there yourself.

Get to Your Ideal Size and Enjoy Life More

Losing weight most likely has been one of your major lifetime projects. Certainly it has taken time and energy. You've learned about nutrition and various diets and food systems. You've succeeded at times and failed most of the time. You may have worked at your weight issues endlessly and worried thousands of hours about your size, your eating, and your behaviors. As you get to your ideal size, you will free up time and energy that can be used more constructively.

Having a weight issue takes time. It takes time to worry about what the scale is going to read and what you can or cannot eat at each meal and snack. It takes time to figure out what clothing will fit on that particular day and how to make yourself look thin even when you aren't. Moreover, it's a drag to go and find one more diet, one more exercise scheme, or one more oddball potion that perhaps will work.

Lose Weight, Find Time

What would happen if much of your weight-management time and energy were put into more uplifting, positive, and satisfying activities? What would happen if you didn't need to constantly diet or worry whether your clothes will fit? How would your life change?

Here's a short quiz to take. Write down your honest answers:

 ◆ How many times a day do you think about your weight?

   _____

   _____

- How often do you step on the scale every week?

  _____

  _____

- How much time do you spend thinking about which foods are "okay"?

  _____

  _____

- How much time do you spend figuring out how to dress in ways that hide your weight?

  _____

  _____

- How often do you feel guilty for eating a particular food?

  _____

  _____

- How many times have you wondered what others thought about your size?

  _____

  _____

- How many hours in your lifetime have you stood looking in the mirror examining your hips and thighs?

  _____

  _____

- Do you think someone who has naturally thin habits spends his or her time doing these things?

  _____

  _____

- What would you rather be doing with your time and energy?

  _____

  _____

Your weight management won't be one of the most significant contributions you make in your life. Your size will not be written about in your obituary. You have more important things to do in life than deal with a weight issue. So make this the last time you put energy and effort into weight loss. Now is the time to get over the issues and get on with your life.

Thinspiration

Make a list of what you would do if you were already at your ideal size. Then either do these things or make plans to do them.

Mastering Your Weight

You are the only person who can master your body's weight. Whether you choose to lose weight in a group or alone, only you get to vote on your size. You determine your success. No one else can do it for you.

By mastering your eating and your weight, you …

◆ Understand your body and its needs.

◆ Know which foods and nutrition work best for you.

◆ Do exercises that make you feel good and look good.

◆ Understand your individual metabolism and how to enhance it.

◆ Stay at your ideal size throughout your lifetime.

◆ Sensuously enjoy food and eating.

◆ Remain in charge of your eating, your size, and your weight.

◆ Set a good example for your children.

Thinspiration

Affirm your life's purpose. Dieting isn't it and neither is overeating. If you aren't sure what it is, pretend you know. Tell yourself, "I am now fulfilling my life's purpose."

The Least You Need to Know

◆ The number of overweight and obese people has reached national epidemic proportions.

◆ By getting to your ideal size, you will improve your health and reduce health risks associated with being overweight and obese.

◆ Generally speaking, women who are at their ideal size earn more income than women who are overweight.

◆ You can begin to enjoy the benefits of looking good and feeling good right now.

◆ As you master your weight, you will free up your energy for more creative and productive pursuits.

Your Ideal Size Is Within Your Reach

In This Chapter

◆ Internal and external barriers to weight loss

◆ What prevents weight loss

◆ Predispositions to being overweight

◆ Changing your weight-loss assumptions

Why is weight loss so difficult? You tackle many problems every day that seem much more challenging—your job, family life, budgets, even just driving a car through traffic. What makes shedding inches and keeping them off so prone to failure?

You already have a weight-loss history of what works and doesn't work for you. You probably also have some prejudices that may not be valid. In this chapter, we give you fresh insights about yourself, both physical and mental. You'll learn to approach losing weight realistically and to determine what can be changed, what can be enhanced, and what needs to be accepted.

Death, Taxes, and Body Shape

Just as death and taxes are inevitable, some aspects of your body condition are inevitable, too. You cannot change them. They can seem like barriers to achieving your ideal size, but they don't have to be. They are as follows:

◆ Aging

◆ Genetics

◆ Hormones

◆ Menopause (for women)

◆ Middle-age spread (for both men and women)

◆ Childbirth (for women)

The Aging Weight Myth

There is a popular myth about aging and weight that goes like this: As you get older, you get bigger. The good news is that it *is* a myth. You do not have to get bigger as you age. There are plenty of older people with great bodies who enjoy eating and stay at their ideal size. Remember, all you need is one example of it not being true to know that it doesn't need to be true for you.

Does age affect body size and shape at all? Of course. In general, as we age, our metabolism naturally slows down. A slower metabolism means we burn calories slower. This means that eating less food will help to avoid weight gain. But with the exercise and physiological knowledge available today, we also know how to boost metabolism through strength training and even through eating well. The good news is that you can keep your metabolism high throughout your life and keep your ideal size.

Your Genes Don't Come from a Designer

You'll have to be content with designer jeans. The genes passed down from your ancestors through your biological parents are yours forever, good and bad. You cannot change your genetics. (Yes, researchers are seeking the "fat" gene, but they still haven't found one that absolutely predicts obesity.) We prefer to treat our genetics as a given, but we can learn to make the most of what we've been given.

An old adage tells us: If your parents and relatives are overweight, you will also be overweight. If you come from a "large" family, this can seem to be true. However, think back for a moment to how your family ate. What size portions did they expect you to eat? Were you required to clean your plate before you got a treat, meaning dessert? Did the family center all celebrations around food and lots of it? Were you taught at an early age to seek out food for solace, celebration, and reward? Maybe it's not your genetics dictating your size but your family's attitude toward food and eating.

> **Body of Knowledge**
>
> Some aspects of heredity affect your body shape, but your genes alone can't make you fat. Heredity is just one of many factors that affect your shape and size.

It appears that behaviors in "fat" families are more likely to predict overweight offspring than genetics. For now, know that you can learn new eating habits. You can leave food on your plate, you can become a picky eater, and you can send your leftover food right down the garbage disposal. Isn't that what a garbage disposal is for?

You can relearn how to eat and how to approach food. In Chapter 27, you will learn how to eat at family gatherings and have fun without overindulging ... all while staying at your ideal size.

Aagh! Those Raging Hormones!

Hormones often get the blame for everything from obesity to thick thighs. Have you ever said to yourself, "If it weren't for my hormones, I would be able to lose this weight?" You are right in part, but only in part. Hormonal systems that are out of balance can wreak havoc on your weight-loss dreams. You could experience a slower metabolism, weight gain around your midsection, and water retention, to name a few of the possible outcomes.

You have considerable power, however, to change your hormonal balance. A combination of proper and delicious nutrition, specific exercises (such as the five Tibetan exercises in Part 4), and plenty of sunshine on a regular basis can help keep your hormones in balance and free up excess stored fat.

You may have hormonal imbalances due to surgical removal of glands such as the thyroid or ovaries. Medications can aid your body in getting necessary hormones. Be sure you are getting enough but not too much. Work with your doctor to adjust your dosage so that you feel your best and have the most energy possible. Be sure to include the recommendations for nutrition, exercise, and sunshine given in this book to keep your hormones in balance.

> **Lean Lingo**
>
> **Hormones** are made within the body to stimulate and regulate cellular and glandular functions.

Hormones definitely affect your weight, but you are not stuck with "bad" hormones. You can do something to balance and energize them.

Menopause Isn't a Menace

As a woman gets to the age of about 50 (give or take), she goes through the change of life, or menopause. This process starts as early as age 30 with *perimenopause*. Her body changes in many ways because her production of estrogen slows down. Her menstrual periods cease, metabolism slows down, and her skin gets thinner.

Unfortunately, plenty of myths about menopause abound, such as menopause being a time when a woman can expect to gain weight. As inevitable as menopause is, it doesn't have to go hand in hand with weight gain. Yes, some women do gain weight at this time of life, most often because their metabolism has slowed way down and they are eating the same amount of food as they did at age 25. Of course this leads to weight gain.

Lean Lingo

Perimenopause is the 10 to 12 year transition leading up to menopause. During this time the body's hormone production slows down.

But if a woman eats just the amount of food that her body needs for fuel, eats nutrient-packed foods, and exercises for both strength and stamina, she can stay at her ideal size with ease.

In other words, menopause is a fact of life. It is not an excuse for being overweight.

That Useless Spare Tire

Men tend to have "spare tires" around their waist come middle age. All the crunches at the gym don't seem to help much. In fact, a man can have terrifically strong stomach muscles and still have a larger waist and midsection.

The spare tire is predominately caused by stress. Adrenaline is the "fight or flight" hormone you excrete during your stress reaction to normal daily events such as driving, working, and so on. The more stress you experience, the more adrenal hormones your body excretes. One of the adrenal stress hormones, cortisol, causes the body to store fat specifically around the waist. So the more stress, the more cortisol production, the more waist. Can this be changed? Yes, in several ways: through eating nutritiously so that you get plenty of stress-busting nutrients, by doing those crunches with complementary stretching, and by decompressing everyday. Yes, that means relaxing.

When "Baby Fat" Isn't on the Baby

Many women complain they never lost the weight they gained during pregnancy. Of course, a woman naturally weighs more during pregnancy and even up to a year after childbirth. A woman is biologically programmed to gradually release her "baby" weight during the first year after birth. Some women, however, don't lose the weight. The baby weight stays on. This can be caused by hormones and also because the women continue to eat as they did when pregnant.

Weighing more during pregnancy is a fact of life. Not being able to lose the "baby" fat doesn't have to be. The situation can be remedied. Your weight is not and never will be a lost cause. Your youthful shape can return just as it has for many other women. By using the nutritional guidelines in Part 3 of this book, you will be able to give your body the support it needs.

But I Love Food!

Yes, you do love food. Hooray! Biologically, you are designed to love food. By eating food, you sustain your life. Food is essential for your well-being, health, and the very survival of the species. Practically everyone loves food. Some food lovers are at their ideal size and some aren't, but confusion about your love of food could be getting in the way of reaching your ideal size. Do any of the following sound familiar?

If It Weren't for Chocolate

If it weren't for chocolate, I would be able to lose weight.

Chocolate is delicious and enticing. It tastes good. It makes me feel good.

The good news is that chocolate is good for you. Chocolate contains plenty of healthy antioxidants and nutrients. The fat content of chocolate provides energy. The bitter and sweet taste is wonderful. Purists may argue that it doesn't belong in a perfect diet, but we are looking for success and a way of eating that lets you have a well-balanced and healthy diet. So enjoy your chocolate—carefully.

Thinspiration

You don't have to give up your chocolate to lose weight. Learn how to eat it slowly and savor every taste sensation. You don't want to completely deny yourself the foods you love because it could lead you to binge out later.

If It Weren't for (You Fill in the Blank)

If it weren't for sugar, bread, butter, steak—you name it—I would be able to lose weight.

Weighty Warning

If you are allergic to any food, you must not eat it because you will get bad results. One of these side effects could easily be weight gain. Symptoms of allergies can range from indigestion, constipation, and/or diarrhea to hives, coughing, and difficulty breathing. If you suspect that you have a food allergy, check with a doctor who specializes in allergies.

Perhaps you have read that certain foods can make you fat, and you believe they contribute to your weight problem. You will learn as you read through this book that any food can make you fat and any food can make you thin, depending on how you eat it.

The good news is that there aren't evil foods. You can eat all foods and enjoy them and get to your ideal size. This doesn't mean you have permission to overeat these foods or to binge on them. Just learn to eat them normally, enjoy them, and let them give you nutrition, pleasure, and energy, which is what food is for.

If It Weren't for Fast Food

Let's face it. Fast food is part of our lives. It is quick, easy, inexpensive, and can sustain us, at least temporarily. Even with the ongoing concern of experts about the poor nutritional content of fast food and the high fat content, you can eat fast food once in a while and lose weight. "Once in a while" is the operative phrase here. In Chapter 26, we will show you how to eat at fast-food restaurants while getting to your ideal size.

Thinspiration

One of the wonderful things about losing weight is that you lose weight by eating, not by avoiding food or starving yourself. Your love of food and enjoyment of it can propel you to your ideal size. What a delight—the very thing that caused your weight gain is the very thing that will bring you success.

Other People and Your Eating

Other people in your life can seem to derail your weight-loss success. Perhaps you have thought that if you didn't have them around, especially at mealtime, you could easily master your weight. The reality, though, is this: Those people *are* part of your life. You can be thin regardless of your relationships with others, and in Chapter 27 we tell you how.

Cooking and Your Eating

You may be cooking meals for a family, including growing children with racecar metabolisms. They can consume masses of spaghetti and never gain an ounce. You not only have to cook for them and eat with them, you are in agony while you watch them devour food.

You can master this situation. The basic guideline is this: Eat the same foods they eat, just not the same quantity. Yes, you can enjoy pizza. You do not need to eat special foods or make a big deal with your family about your diet. You can confidently eat with them and lose weight.

Eating and Your Relationships

If only I didn't have to eat with my spouse.

If only I weren't in a relationship.

If only I were in a relationship.

If only I didn't have to feed my children.

Actually, none of these statements has much to do with what or how you eat, but you might think they do. If you're trying to keep up with another person bite for bite, forkful for forkful, it will not be a "losing" situation.

The late comedian Flip Wilson, imitating a child, would get laughs with his "The devil made me do it!" excuse for being bad. It didn't work for the child, and it won't work for you. We doubt someone is opening your mouth and force-feeding you, so forget trying to place blame elsewhere.

You can learn the skills to eat with others and lose weight at the same time. The simple rules for eating to lose weight are the same regardless of whom you eat with. As you learn to enjoy eating again, you'll rediscover the joys of eating with others—the camaraderie, the interesting conversations, the laughter, the sharing. Dining together is one of the good parts of life. You can feel nurtured and nourished when eating with loved ones.

Thinspiration

Sometimes your friends or spouse subconsciously don't want you to lose weight. Mention your quest to reach your ideal size only to those who will genuinely support you. Otherwise, mum's the word.

Weight Is a Time Issue

It takes time to lose weight. Time as measured in months or years, but also in the time to do what it takes. If you want to know what you love, notice where you put your time. Your priorities are defined by the time you allot for activities. If you don't take the time to lose weight, it isn't a high enough priority.

Remember, worrying about your weight takes time, too. If you devote time now to reaching your ideal size, you'll save time in the long run.

Body of Knowledge

Here's a time guideline to attaining your ideal size. Figure that it takes about two to three months to lose a dress size or belt size. You may lose your weight faster, but use this guide for planning.

Exercise, Time, and You

I don't have enough time to exercise.

No one has time to exercise, do they? Who has time to take off during a busy day and spend 30 to 45 minutes sweating and huffing and puffing? You do. How do we know? Because we know this: If exercise is important to you, you will find a way. If you have enough time to watch just one television show, you have time to exercise.

Besides, exercise isn't about time; it's about love. The love of health, well-being, energy, and vitality. It's about commitment—your commitment to living at your ideal size. You know this.

Cooking, Time, and You

Few people have enough time anymore to cook beautiful meals, so make delicious meals that feature simplicity and good nutrition. Getting the nutrition you need to lose weight doesn't require lots of time cooking. It requires thoughtfulness and care. Having time to cook is not a requirement for losing weight.

Fortunately, you don't have to enjoy cooking to lose weight. It makes no difference whether you cook at home, have others cook for you, eat out, or take something home. Your size is independent of your attitude toward cooking. You can avoid cooking and still get to your ideal size. How? As an example, you can eat raw, fresh foods. You can purchase healthy, ready-made foods from delicatessens and salad bars. Most grocery stores have interesting takeout sections.

Cook stunning meals if you want, but don't sweat it if you and the stove are not on a first-name basis.

> ### Body of Knowledge
>
> With all the information that bombards you about foods, it's no surprise that you might be confused about what to eat. If you tried to follow the combined recommendations of every diet book and nutritionist, you would go crazy—and probably gain weight! In this book, you'll learn about the varied and delicious foods you can eat while getting to your ideal size. Remember, no food is evil.
>
> Be assured that you can find foods you love that will aid you in meeting your weight goals.

Medical Conditions

If you have a medical condition that gets in the way of losing weight, you must learn how to make the best of your health situation. Certain medical conditions can definitely slow down your weight loss, but they don't need to stop or thwart your efforts.

Low Thyroid

An underactive thyroid gland can suppress your metabolism and keep your weight on. Your best bet is to fine-tune your dosage of thyroid medication with your doctor's assistance. If you suspect that your thyroid is out of balance, make sure your doctor assesses all aspects of your thyroid production:

- T3, which is the stronger of the two key hormones produced by the thyroid gland and also produced from the conversion of T4.

- T4, which is the primary hormone produced by the thyroid gland.

- TSH, which is the hormone produced by the pituitary gland that stimulates the thyroid gland. Measurement of TSH is considered a primary way to diagnose thyroid disorders.

Some people respond better on a combination of T3 and T4; some do fine on T4 alone.

Some clients do best on regular prescription meds for thyroid support. Others do best with natural thyroid medication such as Armour.

Daily exercises help to balance your hormones. Be sure to take 5 to 10 minutes every day to do the Tibetan exercises in Part 4.

Hormone Replacement Therapy

If you're using some form of hormone replacement therapy (HRT) to ease the symptoms of menopause, you may feel that it's causing you to gain weight—and it could be, because one of the side effects is a change in weight (either weight gain or weight loss). Ask your doctor to check your dosage to help your weight stabilize. Your doctor might also add some testosterone to your prescription because this may aid in lowering weight and also increasing sex drive.

> **Thinspiration**
>
> Look into other forms of HRT if you are not satisfied with your current prescription. You might prefer natural hormone compounding, which is done at specialty pharmacies. Also talk with your physician about trying estrogen and progesterone creams because they could remedy weight gain.

Hormone replacement therapy is serious stuff, so approach HRT with caution and learn as much as you can about it. Ask your doctor and go to the library to learn about the latest research. Find the methods, whether natural or prescription, that best ease your menopausal symptoms. Make sure you are comfortable with your choice.

Once you have your dosage adjusted correctly, you can lose weight through your efforts to increase your metabolism. Do this with cardio and strengthening exercises and by eating foods as recommended in the nutrition chapters in Part 3.

Some Medications

Several medications can prevent weight loss or cause you to gain weight. Steroids are the trickiest. They virtually always cause weight gain. Even asthma inhalers have enough steroids to slow or stop your progress. Talk with your doctor and ask him or her to suggest alternatives to your current steroid medications. Also ask what you can do to ease off them.

Some psychotropic and antiseizure drugs can also affect your weight. Most often these cause weight loss, but some (such as Depakote) can cause weight gain. Again, ask your doctor to work with you to find one that does not affect your weight.

Pain

Chronic pain can inhibit your desire to exercise. If you are in continual pain from injuries or arthritis, you could also be using food to soothe the pain. Be sure you make other choices for pain relief. Certainly, it can be difficult to do much exercise with severe or chronic pain, but it is possible to do *some* exercise. Get the assistance of a physical therapist or a specialist to find exercises that are healing for you.

Whenever individuals become inactive, for whatever reason, their body needs less food than before. Often people do not adjust their food intake when they become inactive, and they gain weight. If you are currently inactive, be sure you reduce the amount of food you are eating to accommodate your inactivity and the resulting slower metabolism. You will have this slower metabolism until you are able to establish a new exercise routine.

Low Blood Sugar

Low blood sugar happens when your blood sugar drops fast and catches you unaware. At such times, you may experience headaches, nausea, irritability, crankiness, and a lightheaded feeling. You also get heavy-duty cravings for food—any kind of food and lots of it.

Low blood sugar can result in bingeing and in overeating sweet, starchy foods such as cookies, cakes, crackers, and breads. The key to tackling a low-blood-sugar condition is to eat enough protein and fat at meals. Plus, you should keep snacks around—in your handbag or desk—and eat them when you suddenly feel like you are running on empty. By using the nutritional advice in this book, low blood sugar can become an aspect of your past and not your present.

Diabetes

Diabetes and weight gain share an unfortunate symbiotic relationship. Sixty-seven percent of adults with type 2 diabetes have a BMI of 27 or higher. Type 2 diabetes is often called *adult onset diabetes* because a person is not born with it; rather, you develop it as an adult. People who are overweight or obese are at higher risk of developing this chronic disease. If for no other reason, you should get your weight down to reduce your risk of having this difficult health condition.

Type 2 diabetics who regulate their blood-sugar levels with diet and not with insulin can often more easily reach their ideal size. If you are using insulin to control blood-sugar levels, approach any weight-loss program carefully with close monitoring of your blood-sugar levels. That way, you will avoid insulin levels that are too high. Too much insulin in the body can

Weighty Warning

The rate of type 2 diabetes in the United States is skyrocketing, partially due to the increase in obesity. Over 15.6 million adults—or 8 percent of the U.S. population—have type 2 diabetes. If you already have type 2 diabetes, the closer you get to your ideal size, the more likely it is that your health will improve. Even if you don't have diabetes, reaching your ideal size will lower your risk.

cause weight gain. Insulin is one of the body's hormones that causes weight gain when the body has too much.

Birth Control Pills

Birth control pills have been known to cause weight gain—sometimes a little, sometimes a lot—in many women. Fortunately, the hormone dosage in today's birth control pills is lower than ever before and should not be a big factor in weight gain. With that said, however, you could still be gaining weight by using them. If this is the case, talk with your doctor to find a formula that reduces weight gain for you.

The birth control shots and systems that last for three months at a time are more problematic. They can wreak havoc with your body and add on the pounds. Think carefully about whether the three-month formulations are worth the weight. Yes, they are convenient, but are they necessary for you? Find another method if you are battling an increase in weight while using this method.

You Can Master These Weight-Loss Barriers

Certain barriers to weight loss are easy to change. Doing your part from a lifestyle point of view can work wonders. In fact, sometimes making only one change can assist you in shedding pounds.

Enjoy Your Beauty Rest

Are you getting enough vitamin ZZZZ? You need adequate sleep. If you are deprived of sleep regularly, you will struggle to get to your ideal size. Remember the saying "If you snooze, you lose"? Well, hooray! With weight loss, it's true! Research has shown that if you don't snooze, you gain.

Figuring out how much sleep you need is the question. You require basically the same amount of sleep per night every night. Chances are, the amount you need has remained fairly constant throughout most of your life. You probably need somewhere between six and nine hours of sleep every night.

Don't fret if your sleep needs are on the high end. It's not a "badge of honor" to get by on less sleep. This "getting by" attitude is fattening. During sleep, your body relaxes and releases fat. Without enough sleep, your body will hoard fat just in case it has to run on a lack of sleep and rest for days on end.

Plan your life so that you get the sleep your body requires. It will help you reach your ideal size. Yes, some nights you won't get enough sleep, but make them infrequent. Remember, those thin jeans are going to feel so good when they finally fit.

> **Thinspiration**
>
> Here is one way to tell how much sleep you need. Not everyone needs the same amount of sleep. Go to bed before 11 P.M. on a night when you do not have to awaken at a specific time the next day. Don't set the alarm clock. Wake up naturally. Make a note of how many hours you slept. Do this again the next night and the next. The right amount for you will tend to be the average of those last two nights. Yes, it could even be nine hours or more. That's okay. Try to get this amount of sleep every night.

Too Much Fight or Flight Adds Pounds

Living a life of continual high stress will keep you fat and can actually increase your weight. Adrenaline is our friend when we need it for emergencies, but it was never intended to be tapped on a day-to-day basis to deal with traffic, anxiety, work-related issues, and deadlines. If you live with stressful deadlines, a high-stress job, a frantic daily commute, and so forth, losing weight will be an uphill battle … and another source of stress!

Adrenaline is a valuable primitive hormone. When this "fight or flight" hormone is on full alert and is ready to give you the extra energy boost to protect life and limb, your body does not release weight. Instead, it hoards its fat supply so that you have the energy you need to "escape from a woolly mammoth" or fight for your life. In fact, when your adrenaline rush is sustained for long periods of time, the body actually stores extra fat to ensure that your energy supply stays high for months, even years.

Your best choice for dealing with continual adrenaline rush is to schedule time periods when you simply relax. Don't run errands, paint the bedroom, or clean out the garage. Instead, snuggle on the sofa with a good read. Rent funny movies and enjoy some laughs. Give yourself the luxury of really resting, and by the next morning, you may just find that your jeans are looser.

> **Thinspiration**
>
> Ever wonder why you sometimes lose weight on vacation? It could be that your body is off the adrenaline rush long enough to release fat stores it doesn't need. If you vacation infrequently, make a habit of taking a whole day off whenever you can. Then do nothing productive. Amazing, isn't it? Thin and lazy sometimes go together!

The Dark Side of Caffeine

A good cup of coffee is certainly a delight and, for some people, is pretty much a necessity for getting the day started. Perhaps you even drink a cup or two mid-afternoon to

Thinspiration

If you change your morning coffee ritual, you may find yourself getting thinner. Have breakfast with your wakeup cup of coffee. Include some protein, even if it's dinner leftovers. This takes some getting used to. You will love the results.

perk up from an energy slump. The same could be said for tea, caffeinated soda, and diet sodas. Caffeine is tricky. It can prevent you from losing weight and can contribute to weight gain.

How can this be? Caffeine has no calories. But calories are not involved here. Caffeine stimulates the pancreas to, in a sense, overproduce insulin. Insulin is one of the body hormones that cause the body to store fat.

Does this mean you should never have a cup of coffee again? Not really. You don't need to give up caffeine, but you could benefit by changing the way you drink caffeinated beverages. The simple rule of thumb is this: Have your caffeinated beverage *with* a meal, not before a meal or all by itself. (By the way, putting cream and sugar in coffee or tea does not count as a meal.) By having food with your beverage, the insulin is not overproduced; it is more balanced.

It is also perfectly fine to give up caffeine entirely. Plenty of people do. They seem to function fine, although their caffeinated friends find this hard to believe. If you want to get off coffee or caffeine, you can wean yourself off slowly or go "cold turkey." In either case, expect to be physically uncomfortable for a while. The most common reactions are lethargy and headaches. They go away after several days to a week.

Allergies Add Pounds

Eating foods that you are allergic to or sensitive to will work against your best efforts at weight loss. If you're allergic to a food or are highly sensitive to it and you go ahead and eat it anyway, you will pay the price. When you ingest a known allergen, the body gets defensive. It uses several strategies for dealing with allergens: It bloats. It refuses to digest. It might push the food through the digestive tract too quickly. It creates mucous to prevent the food from being absorbed in the intestines. It can wad the food into a ball in your bowel and refuse to dispel it. The body does many things with such a food—except use it for nutrition.

Many foods that cause allergies and sensitivities are common foods that are widely available and seem to be in everything edible. The most difficult to eliminate from your diet include wheat, corn, soy, and dairy products.

If you suspect that you are allergic to a specific food, you can get verification from a skin test given at an allergist's office. In the meantime, give up the food. Some chiropractors also have tests for food sensitivities.

A Little Taste of Sweet

If you make a habit of sipping on sweet liquids—even artificially sweetened ones—throughout the day, you may have difficulty losing weight. Ditto eating mints or bits of candy throughout the day. This isn't really about the calories you ingest; its more about how the sweet taste works with the digestive system.

When the tongue tastes something sweet, the body assumes that it's going to be receiving food and nutrition. It then begins to store the food it is currently digesting, turning that food into fat. After all, the body won't need the energy from the food already in the digestive process if more is on the way. The digestive system doesn't know that it's only going to get a bit of something sweet. It just does as it's programmed—it stores fat.

So, how are you going to drink sweet-tasting liquids like juice or a beverage sweetened with sugar or an artificial sweetener? Have them with meals or with a real snack. A healthy snack is food that you eat intentionally every few hours between regular meals. What about the candy in the jar on your desk or the mints in your purse? Eat them as a real snack, not as a mindless activity. Eating sweets all day long is never a good idea. You will learn more about how and what to eat in Part 3 of this book.

Fortunately, you don't need to be stuck with an impossible weight issue. Today, with medical advances and common sense, there are excellent solutions for tough weight-loss concerns.

> **Thinspiration**
>
> Sip on water during the day as an alternative to sipping on sweet drinks. Sweet drinks, including all diet drinks, confuse the body. Water has terrific therapeutic and health benefits. Your body loves water.

The Least You Need to Know

- ♦ Virtually all body conditions that prevent weight loss can be remedied.
- ♦ Review your reasons for not being able to lose weight and resolve to either correct them or let them go.
- ♦ Do what is necessary to clear up any body conditions that have kept your weight on.
- ♦ Work with your health professionals to correct medical conditions.

3

Choosing Your Ideal Size

In This Chapter

◆ Choosing the size that feels best to you

◆ Using your favorite jeans as a weight benchmark

◆ Selecting your ideal clothing size based on your body frame

◆ Mom's old-fashioned recipe for knowing your ideal weight

◆ Measuring your body fat percentage and BMI

◆ Establishing your attainable goals

You have embarked on a journey to lose weight and get to your ideal size. You need to know your destination. Where do you want to end up? What size will mark the end of your journey? When you select your ideal size, remember that if you don't like it when you get there, you can choose a different size.

Your ideal size is the size that feels the best, at which you have the most energy, the best health, and the highest self-confidence and self-esteem. In this chapter, you will learn several methods for determining your ideal size. We recommend simple strategies but also have included the preferred medical ways to select your size.

Beware the Scales

Thank goodness *scales* are finally out of favor. More and more people and professionals understand the limitations of scales and are finding other methods for weight management.

A scale doesn't really tell you much that you don't already know, but for a perfectly harmless device in itself, a scale sure can alter a person's moods. If you get on a scale in the morning and have lost a pound, you can feel great about yourself all day. Inside, however, you may be wondering why it wasn't two pounds. If you have stayed at the same weight as the day before, you are doing fine, but on second thought not all that well. If the scale reads more than yesterday, you feel like a failure, get depressed, and question the validity of your diet and your self-discipline. You will probably also question the accuracy of the scale! By the end of the day, you can descend into a dire sense of failure that cries out for food, glorious food, to soothe your lowered sense of self-esteem.

Lean Lingo

A **scale** is a device that measures a person's specific gravity in relation to the earth. This reading, usually in pounds, indicates a person's weight. It does *not* tell you what size you are.

Body of Knowledge

A cubic inch of muscle weighs more than a cubic inch of fat. Every cubic inch of fat you release and every cubic inch of muscle you gain will make you look thinner, although your weight may not go down.

Scales scientifically measure your specific gravity in relationship to the earth. That's all. They do not tell you how you look or how much body fat you have. They don't measure what's truly going on inside your body. They only measure your weight at a very specific point in time; they tell you nothing about how you fit into your clothes. But try explaining that logic to a person who compulsively visits the scale six to eight times a day.

A woman who has plenty of healthy muscle mass may appear to be the same size as a woman who has a high percentage of body fat. Who weighs more? The first woman weighs more because muscle weighs more than fat. As you do the strength-training exercises in this book to increase your muscle tone and shape, you could end up weighing more than your goal—and looking better than your goal.

One middle-aged male client, Bill, came to his fifth class session delighted that he needed to purchase a new belt. He had lost about 5 to 6 inches from his waist, but he lamented that he hadn't lost any weight at all. What happened? Bill's new exercise regime and eating patterns resulted in lost inches. Many inches. The weight on the scale was not relevant. He was already at the *size* he wanted.

It might feel scary to not step on the scale daily. Get over it. If the scale is too tempting, put it in cold storage and haul it out once a year for an annual "weigh-in."

Thinspiration

Jockeys, wrestlers, and boxers are among the few professionals who must get on a scale. Many of them hate it, too. Fortunately, there are other ways to measure your weight-loss progress. Get rid of your scale.

How Do Your Jeans Fit?

Jeans are rather unforgiving. They don't have an elastic waistband (at least, we hope they don't). They aren't made from some stretchy knit fabric designed to let you grow unhindered and unobserved. They are denim, rugged and classic denim. They don't budge for your bulges.

Do you have a favorite pair of jeans that you've saved because they once fit? Do you secretly long for the day when you can zip them up comfortably and know you look great? Save those jeans. They are your benchmark for how you are doing with your weight loss. Keep them for the rest of your life.

Now that you're heading toward your ideal size, try on your old favorite jeans every month or so. The jeans cannot lie. They're always the same size. As you progress toward your ideal size, you will easily see the progress you are making. When you finally fit into them, it's a real "hurrah!" moment, one you will savor and use for continual inspiration.

Using the jeans method for determining your ideal size means you don't need to weigh in. Of course, it's not a scientific measurement. Do you care? If you need a target number, you may need another measuring stick. But many people who are already thin use this method to stay at their ideal size. The instant their jeans are tight, they are careful about food intake for a couple of days or weeks until their jeans once again fit comfortably.

Jeans make you feel sexy. They are youthful, fun, and speak loudly and proudly of your weight-loss success.

What's in a Size?

Clothing sizes are an imprecise but highly effective guide to measuring your weight-loss success. If you're a woman, pick a dress size that you would like to wear. If you

Thinspiration

Whatever ideal size you choose, affirm you are that size frequently throughout your day. Say, "I now wear a size (insert your ideal size)." Say it even if you aren't at that weight yet. This may sound nuts to you. That's okay. Say it anyway. Affirm your ideal size as often as you think about it. This activity will propel you toward your goal.

want to shop the size-8 racks, make them your target and imagine yourself doing just that. Go for it. You may find yourself picking a smaller dress-size goal once you've reached your first one.

One of our class participants, Marian, who is in her early 50s, made up a mantra that she said to herself often, "It's never too late to be an 8." Upon reaching that goal, she wrote yet another mantra with the assistance of her son Michael, "It's the kicks to be a 6." Within several months, Marian was buying size 6 shorts—a size she never thought possible when she was a size 12.

Women usually think of size in terms of dress size, men in terms of their belt size. So, fellows, if you want a waist size of 34, 36, or whatever, select the one that feels best to you.

Using the select-a-size method to choose your ideal size is not particularly scientific, but it's a good measure for how you look—and no scale is needed. It works for many people.

Before you select your ideal size for certain, you need to learn about your frame size.

The Frame You Were Born With

The size of your body frame gives a good indication of what clothing size would work best for you. Body frames come in three sizes: small, medium, and large. A person's frame size doesn't change over a lifetime, just as the color of one's eyes doesn't change. Regardless of the size of your frame, you can get to a clothing size that feels good to you.

Body of Knowledge

Here is how to determine your body frame size. Take your dominant hand. Encircle the wrist of your nondominant hand with the middle finger and thumb. If your middle finger and thumb overlap, you have a small frame. If they just touch, you have a medium frame. If they don't touch, you have a large frame.

A woman with a small frame can wear a smaller size because her hipbones are closer together. She could be comfortable at a size 6 or 8, perhaps a 10. With a medium frame, a woman might choose to be a size 8, 10, or 12. With a large frame, perhaps she would choose a size 10, 12, or 14. While a size 14 could sound like a large size to you, we have plenty of clients who look terrific and thin at that size. Your dress size is actually less important than how you look in your clothes and the state of your health at that size.

Hollywood press releases and glamour magazines tell us that some of our favorite movie and television actresses wear a size 0 or 2. You may be wondering how this is possible. Many people who are highly photogenic—think high-fashion models and screen stars—have tiny little faces. Generally speaking, they have very small body frames. Their hipbones are quite close together, and they can wear very small sizes.

These people are genetically unusual—they simply aren't like most of us. Don't worry about it. It's important that you are comfortable and content with the frame size you were born with and make the most of it.

Mother's Rule of Weight

If you're definitely the type who wants to use pounds as your benchmark, try to use weight as just one of your guides to measure your ideal size. And keep it simple. I (Lucy) was surprised to learn that my mother's old-fashioned way for determining if she was overweight is one used by dietitians today. Mom started using her method in the 1950s. Here's how it goes.

For women, take your height and determine how many inches taller you are than 5 feet. For a woman who is 5'8", the answer is 8. Multiply that number by 5 and add it to 100. The total is 140 pounds, her target weight.

Now let's take frame size into account. A small-framed woman who is 5'8" would have a target weight 10 percent less than 140, or 126 pounds. A large-framed woman might be 10 percent more, or up to 154 pounds.

For men, multiply the inches above 5 feet by 6. A 5'11" man would weigh, let's see, $6 \times 11 = 66 + 100 = 166$ pounds (again, plus or minus 10 percent). The weight range for that height is 149 to 182.

Mom's Simple Formula

Your height in inches: _____

Less 60 =   _____

Times 5 for women   _____

Times 6 for men   _____

Added to 100 equals   _____ (medium frame)

Less 10% equals   _____ (small frame)

Add 10% equals   _____ (large frame)

Mother's rule of weight doesn't take into account the amount of muscle a person has. Higher muscle mass could increase the weight on mother's rule by 20 percent or so.

Fat and Muscle Weight Are Quite Different

Another significant measure of body size is body fat percentage. The higher your body fat percentage, the more at risk you are for health issues related to being overweight or obese. When you get your body fat tested at a health club or at the doctor's, the machine gives you a reading of body fat, water, and muscle percentage. All three add up to 100 percent. Assuming that the amount of water weight remains almost constant, the variables are body fat and muscle. The more muscle you have, the less body fat you have (and vice versa). Muscle weighs three times more than fat.

Here are ideal body fat percentages:

Women:	Up to age 20	14–21%
	Age 20 to 50	17–27%
	Age 50+	20–30%
Men:	Up to age 20	9–15%
	Age 20 to 50	14–21%
	Age 50+	19–23%

In body fat measurements, lower is not necessarily better. A person must have at least some body fat to be healthy. Fat pads internal organs such as the kidneys, and it also offers protection against cold weather. For women, the minimum recommended fat percentage is 12 percent. If a woman has less, her menstrual cycles could cease. Men must have a minimum of 5 percent to stay healthy.

As you lose weight and do strength-building exercises, your body fat percentage goes down and your muscle mass increases. This is good because having more muscle gives you the following:

- More physical stamina
- More energy
- A higher metabolic rate
- Better muscle definition
- Less cellulite
- Better shape (for guys, muscle definition; for gals, curves)

- Higher weight as measured on a scale

- Lower risk of diseases associated with being overweight or obese

A high percentage of body fat is not good. More body fat gives you the following:

- Higher risk of diabetes and other diseases associated with being overweight or obese

- Less energy

- A lower metabolic rate

- Inclination to obesity

- A flabby body

Using body fat percentage as a method to measure your ideal size can be misleading. One client, Susie, had a body fat reading of only 19 percent. She wore a size 10. However, her waist was quite thick, and her muscles were so large that she didn't like how she looked in clothes. Her jeans didn't fit. Her body fat percentage was ideal, but she still was a larger size than she wanted. Susie needed to eat differently. Consider using body fat as one measure of your goal but not the only measure.

Thinspiration _____

By doing strength-training exercises for as little as six months at two to three hours a week, a person can reduce his or her body fat percentage by as much as 10 percentage points.

The Professional Choice—BMI

Health and medical professionals use the body mass index (BMI) to determine whether you are overweight or obese. The formula figures both weight and height together but doesn't take into account body fat percentage and muscle mass. To understand BMI, first calculate your own.

Your BMI Calculation

Your weight in pounds ____ × 704.5 = _____
Divide this number by your height in inches = _____
Divide again by your height in inches = _____
This last number is your BMI.

If your BMI is between 18.5 and 24.9, you are in the healthy BMI range. If it is equal to or over 25, you are considered to be overweight. If it is equal to or greater than 30, you are considered to be obese. (If it is below 18.5, you're too skinny and need to get some meat on those bones of yours!)

Having just done the calculation, you know if your BMI makes sense or not for you and your body type. If a person has lots of muscle, he or she can be well into the 25–30 BMI range and not look overweight or be at risk for health issues related to being overweight.

Nutritionists often modify the BMI measurements to take into account different categories of weight and size. The numbers for men are slightly higher than for women.

Women Are:	
Underweight	If BMI is less than 19.1
Ideal weight	19.1 to 25.8
Marginally overweight	25.9 to 27.3
Overweight	27.4 to 32.2
Obese	32.3 to 44.8
Extremely obese	over 44.8
Men Are:	
Underweight	If BMI is less than 20.7
Ideal weight	20.7 to 26.4
Marginally overweight	26.5 to 27.8
Overweight	27.9 to 31.1
Obese	31.2 to 45.4
Extremely obese	over 45.4

If the BMI technique works for you and your body type, you may want to work backward to figure out what weight you need to be to achieve your healthy target BMI.

1. Take your target BMI. (Let's say it is 24.)

2. Multiply the BMI by your height in inches.

3. Multiply again by your height in inches.

4. Divide by 704.5.

This gives you a target weight that you can track on the scale. At least, you can until your muscle mass increases.

Body of Knowledge

Another measurement that professionals use is the waist/hip ratio. Measure your waist at its smallest place and your hips at their widest. Divide your waist measurement by your hip measurement. If the number is nearly 1.0 or greater, you are at greater risk for some health problems such as diabetes, heart disease, and certain kinds of cancer. For a healthy weight, a woman's ratio should be less than 0.80; a man's should be less than 0.95.

Your Attainable Goal

Yes, there are many ways to determine your target ideal size. Test the methods described in the preceding sections. Try them on for size and see which ones fit you the best. We generally recommend that your primary goal should be based on a measurable size, such as jean size, dress size, or belt size. These are measures of how you actually look—to yourself and to others.

Although we are not fond of the bathroom scale, you can consider a weight-based measure if you're so inclined. But if those daily weight fluctuations (and you will have them) cause you to suffer emotional fluctuations, too, just stay off the scale and use your jeans.

Getting your body fat percentage into a healthy range is an admirable goal, too, but you may find only limited benefit from highly precise measurements. Body fat percentage is certainly not something you should measure with great frequency. With a regular routine of moderate strength exercises, you will *know* your body fat percentage is decreasing. You can see—and feel—the new muscle. That's a lot more fun.

With all that said, we strongly encourage you to create your ideal size goal or goals. They are not just destinations on a journey; they are your guideposts along the way. Think of them as "friends," not as enemies. Embrace them with optimism and determination. In Chapters 25 and 26, we will show you powerful ways to win the mental game of weight loss. But for now, simply assume that you will reach your goals.

Here is a place to write down your goals according to the methods you have chosen. We recommend that you include your desired jean size and body fat percentage as two of your weight-loss measurements.

My Weight Loss Goals

My desired jean size _____

My desired body fat percentage_____

My desired dress or belt size _____

My desired BMI _____

My desired weight_____

My desired weight with Mom's method _____

My preferred weight-loss goal is _____ using the _____ method.

The Least You Need to Know

◆ Your ideal size is the one you want to be, the one that gives you the most energy, and the one that feels the best.

◆ All methods for determining your ideal size have advantages and drawbacks.

◆ Select your ideal size using a primary measure and focus on it.

◆ Affirm to yourself often that you are already at your ideal size.

Chapter 4

Stay the Course, Results Will Follow

In This Chapter

- ◆ Tenacity with gentleness is key
- ◆ Changing your attitudes about food
- ◆ Staying on your weight-loss program
- ◆ Right sizing for you and your food

What do you have to show for all the time, energy, and money spent on weight loss in your life? Not much. In fact, you could be larger than ever before. If you aren't larger, perhaps you feel flabbier and more discouraged. You know your efforts haven't produced desired results. What's not working?

A significant part of mastering your weight is conquering the barriers that get in your way. In this chapter, we tell you how to avoid and correct the common pitfalls you could encounter. These include weight loss plateaus, discouragement, and using food to soothe stress and anxiety.

Staying the Course

A good weight-loss system is only as good as your commitment. With a balanced, practical system spiced with common sense, you can be successful. All systems are destined to fail, though, if you fail the system. An effective weight-loss system is one that incorporates the following aspects: how to eat, balanced nutrition, exercise, and attitude. Let's look at what you need to bring to a good weight-loss program for you to win at weight loss.

Tenacity and Patience

Tenacity is the most critical factor for weight loss. In the words of Winston Churchill, "Never, never, never, never, never give up."

Figure that it takes two to three months for a woman to lose a dress size healthfully. Ditto for a man to lose 2 inches of belt size. If you are starting at a size 20 and want to be a size 10, it could take as long as 15 months. Can you hang in there for the long haul?

You could be thinking to yourself, "Fifteen months! By then I'll be almost a year and a half older. Do I have to be larger than I want to be for 15 months?" You know the answer. It's yes. Think of it this way: You will be 15 months older anyway. When you get there, would you rather be overweight or your ideal size?

Thinspiration

If you step on the scale every day and expect to see miraculous weight loss, you will be disappointed. If you must use the scale, limit your visits to once a month.

To reach your goal, you cannot allow yourself to be derailed by stress, depressed emotions, or an off-the-cuff comment from friends or family. Although you want quick results, it's easy to get discouraged when you don't see visible results right away.

Weight loss takes as long as it takes.

Starting the Journey to Your Ideal Size

When you begin a weight-loss program, you are starting a growth process, just like planting a seed. After planting the seed, it needs time to germinate. If you become impatient to see the tiny green plant shoot and decide to dig up the seed to see if it's germinating, you will kill the plant. Germination is the time for patience. As you eat nutritiously and exercise faithfully, you will see some changes, but you cannot reach your weight goal overnight, just as the seed doesn't sprout overnight.

Fruition is when the seed bears flowers and fruit. For you, fruition of your goal is when those jeans fit comfortably. The attainment of your ideal size can take months and perhaps even years from when you begin. Be patient. Good things come to those who persevere and wait.

Thinspiration

Your body is your work of art, right? In the beginning, a painter's efforts are just oil and canvas. But eventually— voilà!—the painter creates a masterpiece. It will take time to turn your body into a masterpiece, too. But you can do it!

Food, Food, Everywhere Food

We are bombarded with weight-loss advertising and news reports about the growing "size" of the population. At the same time, Madison Avenue tries to seduce us with advertising that promotes food and eating. The newsstand formula for selling checkout counter magazines is simple: Picture a luscious-looking dessert and a headline that reads, "Lose 10 pounds in a week." These magazines fuel our national love-hate affair with food and eating.

Fast-food restaurants tantalize us with offers to "supersize" our orders because of the extra "value" we get. Sit-down restaurants serve portions that are big enough for two or three people. We are repeatedly encouraged to assume that big is better … even when it's not.

Supersize meals lead to supersize bodies. These hefty meals offer enough food to feed two, three, or four people. Rather than getting supersize meals, get a right-size meal. Get just enough to meet your body's needs and no more.

Today, food is more widely available and abundant for the average person than at any other time in the history of man, especially in first-world countries such as the United States. This hasn't always been the case. You don't have to go back far in history to find times when food was *not* plentiful. Many people lived in a feast-or-famine environment. When food was plentiful, they ate lots of it because they didn't know where their next meal was coming from. They ate richly whenever they could to store enough fat so that they could make it through the lean times. Today, in our country food is plentiful, but many people eat as their ancestors did—eagerly and anxiously— as if they don't know when they are going to eat again.

Practically any food you could possibly want is available right now within less than an hour's drive of your home. Even if you live away from a city, you can order your

Thinspiration

Give yourself a quiet mental pat on the back each time you stop eating because you've had enough but not too much. Others probably won't notice. Overeating is nothing to brag about.

favorite foods through the Internet and mail-order catalogs. You can't even begin to eat all the food that is available to you.

Think of a T-shirt emblazoned with the saying "So much food, so little time." Hopefully that has not been your food motto. If it has, change it. How about a T-shirt that reads, "I eat all that I need but not more than I need." Or it might have a motto of "I eat plenty but not more than enough." These mottos add an elegance to eating that lets you be in control. It lets you transcend the caveman urge to fill up at every food station on your path through life.

For now, think about right-sizing both your body and your food intake. Plan to take in enough food to stay healthy and active. Plan to stop eating supersize meals before they supersize you.

Nothing Ventured, Nothing Lost

Have you almost given up on losing weight and getting to your ideal size? Has your weight-loss history led you to believe that being thin is only a temporary condition? Are you afraid to lose and gain yet one more time? If so, you are more normal than you might think.

Being afraid of failing at weight loss one more time can be immobilizing. Being immobilized by this fear is almost like giving up on yourself as a person, and you don't want to do that. You may be thinking, "So what's a couple of pounds or a couple more? It absolutely doesn't define who I am as a person. It doesn't speak to my value or my contributions." You are correct. However, it does speak to your interest in your health and your sense of self esteem. The healthier you are, the more you can contribute to yourself and others for many more years.

By using the advice in this book, you can be assured that you are doing what is necessary to give you the benefits you want. You will show yourself and others your courage and interest in being around for the long haul.

Reaching Plateaus

As you lose weight, you may hit a plateau. Your best efforts seem to stall. You stay the same size regardless of what you do. One client, Deborah, went from a size 26 to a size 18 very quickly, within six months. Then she stayed at a size 18 for almost a year before her weight started down again. Deborah had the wisdom to wait it out. She kept to her eating and exercise plans and continued to live normally. Eventually, her body began to release more excess fat, and today she is delighted to be a size 14.

What happens during plateaus? We like to think of them as "still points." Let's compare a plateau in weight loss to water boiling. You put the water into a pot on the stove and turn the heat on high. Not much happens for what seems like a long time (especially if you are watching the pot boil!). During that time, thermal energy is transferred from the burner into the water. As the thermal energy is transferred, the water increases in temperature until it reaches the boiling point. The thermal energy is finally converted into kinetic energy, and you can observe the pot boil.

So it is with weight loss. At the time when nothing seems to be happening, plenty is going on in your body that can't be seen. The body must change a lot as it loses weight. As the body converts fat into energy, the liver detoxifies the by-products and releases them to be excreted as waste products. The body reshapes itself, using up plenty of vitamins, minerals, and trace elements as it does so. The body works extra hard as it releases fat. You should expect that it would rest and regroup from time to time.

Emotionally, plateaus are challenging. You want results and want them fast. Deborah's patience and tenacity pulled her through a year-long plateau. A plateau is the time to stay the course, say aloud your weight-loss affirmations, refine your nutritional and exercise programs, and keep the faith.

Food Is Only Food

Food is excellent for supplying nutrition, energy, and sensory delights, but it does not have magic powers. It can't heal a broken heart. It can't make a skinned knee stop hurting.

People turn to food to do the impossible— to make emotional pain go away, to avoid loneliness, and to improve high-anxiety moments. People want food to solve some basic issues of life. It can't. It has no power. You have the power to do those things.

If you have ever hoped that food would solve things, just remember how disappointed you were when the food failed you. Perhaps you

Thinspiration

Overeating is never the solution, no matter what the problem. It only leads to more problems. Overeating can't heal a broken heart, make you more comfortable at a party, or eliminate stress. All that it can do is add on more pounds.

have returned to food again and again, seeing if things have changed and that somehow food could solve anything.

By now, you absolutely know it can't. But are you still hoping? This kind of hope is terrifically fattening. Give it up. Find wiser ways to solve life's problems.

Food is also not the same as love. Certainly, we prepare food for our families because we love them, but whether they eat the food has nothing to do with whether they are accepting of our love. Ditto for someone preparing food for you. You are not required to eat everything just because someone made it for you. Show your love in many other ways and let food be just food.

Guilt Is a Choice, Not a Requirement

Ever notice how guilt about overeating begets more overeating? Take a binger who is usually overly careful about her food intake. She counts calories or fat grams (or both) and can be seen obsessing over whether to have dressing on her chef salad at lunch.

Every once in while, though, that strong and virtually undeniable urge to overeat surfaces and she gives in. At those times, she forgets about calories and fat grams. She eats heavy foods, laden with all the richness she has been denying herself. At first it feels good, but then it feels awful. Not only is her stomach stuffed and extended, all her careful eating has been ruined. She feels horrible and hates her behavior and herself. She can't understand why she did it. Remorse builds up inside her. The tears come after this seemingly crazy behavior.

So does guilt. This feeling starts eating at her. How could she? What's wrong with her? Bingeing is a bad thing to do. How can she ever atone for this mistake? The guilt wells up inside. Soon she is eating to assuage the guilt. The guilt is layered just like that magnificent torte she inhaled. Guilt for what she did, guilt for ruining her diet, guilt at such bizarre behavior. Guilt at being overweight. Talk about the guilt of the world resting on someone's shoulders.

The more she binges and the more she overeats, the guiltier she feels. Then she eats more to deal with the yucky feelings. Cause and effect become blurred. What is a person to do?

The first step in breaking the guilt-eating syndrome is to forgive oneself. Forgive yourself for all the offenses you thought you did: overeating, bingeing, being fat, being out of control, you name it. As you do this, the guilt releases and you are free and fresh. Then wait until you are hungry and eat normally until your body's hunger is satisfied.

Guilt is a useless, unproductive emotion when it comes to reaching your ideal size. Tell yourself, "It is okay and important to eat. I eat just enough food and not more than my body needs." You'll discover that eating without guilt is a great feeling, one you will enjoy regularly as you gain mastery over your eating habits. Guilt ruins almost all dieting attempts.

> ### Body of Knowledge
>
> In any situation in which you have overeaten, forgive yourself. You simply forgot that you were at your ideal size and that you have mastered your weight and eating. Then wait until you are hungry and eat enough but not too much.

Lucy's Losing Journey

I, Lucy, was a classic yo-yo dieter in college and through my early 30s. I tried many diets and food schemes such as vegetarian macrobiotic eating. I lost weight many times but always regained it. My top weight was 175 or a large size 14. As a heavy-duty binger obsessed with eating and food, I thought I was addicted to sugar and chocolate.

I cried a lot about my weight, and even worse, I never stopped thinking about food and eating. By the time I was finally ready to release my weight issue forever, I most wanted to lose my constant mental obsessing about food and my weight.

By then, having spent a small fortune trying every popular weight-loss program, I began looking for alternative methods. Over a year or two, I read a couple of books, went to several counselors and classes, and finally figured it out. I realized that I could walk away from my weight issue and never return. It was a choice I made.

By using affirmations and visualizations (which are discussed in Chapter 25), I stopped overeating and began to eat normal foods. I forgave myself for all the pain I was causing my loved ones and myself. Within six months I was wearing a size 6, and I have stayed there for over 20 years. I have no idea what I weigh because I don't use scales. My jeans fit. I enjoy food. I eat some sugar and chocolate in moderation along with a nutritionally balanced diet. I seldom eat starches.

I easily maintain my size 6 by doing the same things I did to lose my weight—eating normally, that is, eating only when I was hungry and stopping when I had eaten enough food, before I was full. I exercise about five to six hours a week, doing the

Five Tibetans (see Part 4) and cardio daily, plus two Pilates sessions a week. For recreation, my husband and I go dancing and hiking.

The Least You Need to Know

- Stay the course of your weight-loss program with tenacity, patience, and desire.

- Should you reach a weight-loss plateau, keep on keeping on and doing what works.

- With the vast abundance of food available in the United States, there is no need for you to overeat at any meal.

- Food is not love and can't solve life's problems.

- Guilt is useless and counterproductive when it comes to weight loss.

Part 2

Your Body of Information

Even though we live in the twenty-first century, our bodies basically function the same as the bodies of our caveman ancestors. This bit of trivia may seem unimportant, but it's really quite significant for weight loss. Our bodies digest food in the same way that our ancient ancestors' bodies did, but our diets sure aren't the same.

Your body is biologically programmed to burn food as fuel and store excess food as fat for later use. This part of the book helps you understand the basic primitive nature of your body and how it processes food. You'll learn to appreciate your appetite, really listen to your body's hunger signals, and avoid some of our modern overeating traps.

Some habits that are part of our everyday lifestyles make weight management difficult, but now's your chance to replace them with alternatives that will make you healthier, thinner, and happier.

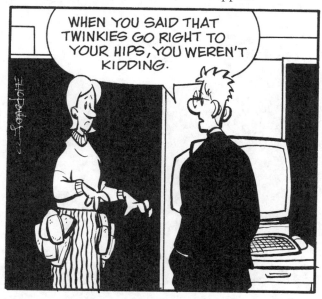

Chapter 5

What Your Body Wants You to Know

In This Chapter

- ◆ Hearing what your body is trying to tell you
- ◆ The actual size of your stomach
- ◆ Eating as your body and stomach direct
- ◆ Eliminating bad eating habits
- ◆ Hearing your body's hunger signals
- ◆ Using a hunger scale to guide your eating

The body is utterly amazing. It takes food in and processes it into energy while extracting nutrients. It manages to excrete what it doesn't need and to store any excess energy supplies as fat. Aaah, there's the rub. Your body's fat-storage system is a natural part of the body's digestive process. It is programmed to add layers of fat, especially when it gets more food than it needs! Now your task is to use up those fat stores and avoid storing even more fat.

If Only Your Body Could Talk

An essential part of losing weight is learning how to listen to your body. We all wish it could just say what it wants. Although it doesn't have an oral language, it does communicate. Certainly, you know when your body hurts because you feel pain. You know when it needs rest because you get the unmistakable cues of nodding off, yawns, and sleepiness. But are you able to clearly hear your body communicate when it is time for you to eat and when it is time to stop eating?

Infants know these signals well. So do animals that live in the wilderness. Most adult humans don't remember the language of hunger and satiation. Infants cry to signal that they need a feeding. Infants know how they are doing by how they feel. If they feel good, everything is fine in their world. If they don't feel good, if something hurts or irritates them, they let mama know right away. By observing an infant cry for food, you can tell that hunger is an actual discomfort. It is felt in the stomach.

Infants also seem to know instinctively when to stop eating. You can tell when they have had enough milk because they simply stop feeding. Midbottle, middrop, it doesn't matter to an infant how much milk is left. Mama may want the infant to drink more milk so that the infant sleeps through the night, but the infant refuses. Why? Because he or she instinctively knows that even one more drop may produce feelings of discomfort. That discomfort is so significant that an infant will not risk the irritation. Besides, he or she is already satisfied.

> **Thinspiration**
>
> Too much of a good thing, even mother's milk, is simply too much. A baby realizes instinctively when it is time to stop feeding. Now is the time for you to relearn this skill.

"Full" Is Not Your Friend

Changing your perception about being *full* could be one of the most critical steps toward reaching your ideal size. Notice that an infant does not keep feeding on milk until he or she is full. Full is actually an uncomfortable feeling. Wanting to get full from eating is an urge that develops later in life due to social pressure and outside messages from family and peers. Infants feed only until they have enough nourishment but not too much. They eat until the hunger urges abate or until their hunger is satisfied and the stomach is comfortable.

> **Lean Lingo**
>
> The feeling of a **full** stomach is a signal that you have eaten too much food. Typically, people who are overweight are accustomed to eating until they are full. Usually this is eating a quantity of food bigger than your fist—give or take.

The good news is that you were once an infant and you knew how to listen to your body's hunger signals.

You have since changed your eating habits to accommodate social norms and emotions, but at the beginning of your life, you ate based on your body's needs. Let's learn how to get closer to those original instincts about food. You may never need to feel full again … and you will be thrilled with the results.

Hunger Is Your Friend

Hunger is good. Hunger is a natural part of your body, and it would be disastrous not to feel hunger. Without the capability to feel hunger, a wild animal would die from starvation. Hunger is a grand thing because it tells us when it is time to eat. Every time you feel true hunger in your stomach, it is time to eat. For some of us, that is three times a day. For some, it could be six times a day. For some, the frequency of feeling hunger pangs can vary from day to day.

It is never a wise practice to do things to avoid feeling hunger. You are supposed to feel hunger so that you can know when it's time to eat to sustain life. You may be thinking that your hunger is out of control. Most often, it isn't out of control; rather, you have either denied or ignored it for so long that its communications are no longer clear. You can trust real stomach hunger.

However, there is a sort of fake hunger. It comes from stress and anxiety, sometimes from appetite stimulants such as alcohol, illegal drugs, or a lack of sleep. The fake hunger is just that. The communication doesn't come from a hunger pang; more likely it comes from the mouth, as in an oral chewing need, or from thirst.

Feeling hunger and understanding how your body communicates hunger are important tools to use in losing weight and staying at your ideal size for life.

How to Feel Hunger

Hunger is a pain, and it is felt somewhere above, below, or behind your belly button. Hunger feels different for different people. For some, it is almost like a muscle contraction. For others, it is an empty or void feeling.

To get acquainted with your hunger, wait to eat until you feel a hunger pang. For most people, it takes about two to five hours after the previous meal to feel some hunger.

> **Body of Knowledge**
>
> Stomach growls are caused by the stomach muscle contracting. When food is in the stomach, the muscles move food through into the small intestine. When your stomach is empty, however, you can hear and feel the "growls." Usually, this is a signal that you are hungry and it is time to eat.

Really pay attention to the feeling of hunger. Identify where the physical feelings are located. Listen intently to any rumbling or growling. Perhaps you are chuckling at the thought of "listening" to your stomach, but learning your own body signals is remarkably powerful.

What Gets in the Way

Listening to your hunger signals is incredibly useful in getting to your ideal size. Unfortunately, many of us have a tough time getting the message because certain conditions block us from "hearing" them. Here are a few of the common blockages:

◆ **Low blood sugar.** If you miss feeling the hunger pang and instead become lightheaded, jittery, irritable, or cranky, go ahead and eat. You could have low blood sugar, which speaks more loudly than hunger pangs, at least at first. When you eat based on the nutritional advice in Part 3—by getting protein, fats, and carbohydrates at every meal—your low blood sugar will lessen, and you can feel your hunger pang better.

◆ **Painkillers.** If you are on painkillers, either prescription or over the counter, you may not be able to feel the sensations of hunger. Other medications, such as antiseizure medications, can also prevent you from feeling hunger. If this is your situation, be sure to read the section "A Fist Full of Food" later in this chapter.

◆ **Nervous stomach.** If you feel anxiety as pain in your stomach, you might mistake the anxiety pain for a hunger pang. If this happens to you, see the section "A Fist Full of Food" later in this chapter.

◆ **Too busy to feel.** If you get so busy that you can shut out the world, most likely you can also shut out your hunger feelings. Set your watch or alarm to ring every hour to remind you to ask your stomach if it is time to eat (that is, if it is hungry).

◆ **No experience.** Perhaps you have ignored your body's hunger communications for most of your life. You may not be able to feel them because you are out of practice. Some people, in fact, never let themselves get hungry. If this is your situation, take time to listen and hear your body's faint and subtle hunger messages. The more you are able to take the time to listen, the louder the messages become. Eventually, you will hear them on an hour-to-hour, day-to-day basis talking to you loud and clear.

Smile when you feel stomach hunger. It is confirming that you haven't been overfeeding it continuously. Then reward it with just the right amount of delicious food.

Satisfaction

As previously mentioned, an infant stops feeding when his or her hunger is satisfied. How does the baby know? The answer is similar to the fable of Goldilocks and the three bears. Goldilocks looked for the porridge, the chair, and the bed that felt just right. The same should be true with your stomach and feeling satisfied. The satisfied stomach isn't a little bit hungry or a little bit full. It feels just right.

Being satisfied is pretty much a nonfeeling. You aren't full, but your stomach hunger pangs have ceased. You have room to take a deep breath. The waistband on your pants doesn't cut into the flesh of your waist. You have enough energy to take a walk or do an activity. You don't feel full, just satisfied.

People who are overweight have become accustomed to eating until they are full. Changing this habit can be extremely difficult. You will learn techniques for monitoring and modifying this behavior at the end of this chapter in the book, but it helps if you face this issue now and face up to your own eating habits.

Weighty Warning

In our culture, when children want to be excused from the dinner table, we often ask, "Are you full?" Change this now to "Did you get enough?" Don't encourage eating until full but to the point of satisfaction.

What Do You Prefer: Full or Satisfied?

Answer the following questions:

1. Do you usually go back for seconds at dinner or lunch? ✓Yes __No

2. Do you "supersize" your meal at fast-food restaurants? __Yes ✓No

3. Do you loosen your belt or change to looser clothes at the end of a meal more than once a month? __Yes ✓No

4. Do you eat a dessert at the end of a meal even when you're satisfied and have had plenty of food? __Yes ✓No

5. Do you regularly drink more than one beer or glass of wine with a meal? __Yes ✓No

6. Do you usually eat everything on your plate, as in being a member of The Clean Plate Club? ✓Yes __No

7. After dinner, do you usually just sit and watch TV or some other sedentary activity? ✓Yes __No

8. Do you eat more than one piece of bread along with everything else on your plate at a main meal? __Yes __No

If you answered "Yes" to more than one or two of these questions, you probably have a habit of eating enough food to feel "full," eating beyond the point of feeling satisfied. As you work toward reaching your ideal size, you will adopt new habits that let you answer "No" to these questions.

Two Simple Rules for Eating Naturally

Eating naturally is eating based on honoring your body's hunger communications. Take a cue from infants who eat only when they are hungry. You only need to remember two broad rules:

- ◆ Only eat when you feel a hunger pang.
- ◆ Only eat enough food to get satisfied, not enough to get full.

Virtually any healthy eating plan or diet program you choose will work if you honor these two key body communications. If you don't honor them, frankly, you should expect to fail.

A Fist Full of Food

Make a fist and observe the size of it. This is about the size of your stomach. Oh dear, you may be thinking, "How did all of that food I ate last night fit into a space so small?" Good question. First, realize that you almost certainly ate more than you needed to feel satisfied. Next, understand that your stomach is a muscle that can expand to accommodate a great amount of food. Just ask anyone who is a binge eater.

Usually, eating an amount of food the size of your fist is enough to get you to feel satisfied ... give or take, based on the day, the weather, the cycles of the moon, and other unspecified mysteries of life and eating! To figure out the amount of food to eat based on comparing it to the size of your fist, you've got to imagine the food in a compressed state. Imagine that the air is taken out of such foods as a salad.

Thinspiration

The only time it is "time to eat" is when the stomach says, "Ouch, feed me." If you aren't hungry—that is, if you do not feel a true hunger pang—don't eat.

Seriously, you can't go wrong eating an amount of food the size of your fist three or four times a day. You certainly won't gain weight. Better yet, you'll start releasing stored fat.

Eating Less Means More Satisfaction

You may be studying the size of your fist right now, already feeling deprived. "That's not much food for me," you could be saying to yourself. You are right, that's not much food, yet it is plenty of food. A fistful is still plenty of food to sustain your life, give you energy, release excess fat stores, look great, feel great, and get healthier.

But what about that deprived feeling you may have, the one that says, "Is this all I get?" Of course, it is always your choice how much you eat, but a fistful of food is all your body needs at a meal. So make sure you eat the most absolutely delicious and nutritious foods and your favorite foods first; otherwise, you won't have room for them. This rule of thumb also applies to buffets, eating out, and parties—every time you are hungry. Be sure to eat slowly so you can savor every morsel of food you eat. The taste lasts longer that way.

Thinspiration

Your stomach can stretch up to six times its normal size when it is stuffed full of food. The amount of food that equals the size of your fist may not seem like very much food. It really is plenty of food. Eat slowly to savor every bite.

Going Against the Body's Natural Flow

Most people who overeat upset the body's designed eating rhythms. Ideally, we only eat when hungry, we stop eating when we have enough, and we let the body digest that food before we have more. Being overweight means eating against the body's best interests.

There are several ways in which overweight people eat that are counterproductive. All of these ways of eating (described in the sections that follow) are harmful to the body's digestive systems and to health. All of them basically ignore the body's hunger signals.

The Continual Feeder

This person always seems to be eating something. The continual eater never gives the body a beginning or ending to a meal. He or she just keeps stoking a machine that has enough to do just digesting what's already in the stomach. The stomach of a continual feeder never gets a rest. Think of watching TV on the sofa with a bag of potato chips. All of a sudden, it seems, the potato chips are gone and the person can't remember eating them. Continual feeders often dislike the feelings of hunger. They avoid hunger feelings by continually feeding.

The Big-Meal Fan

This person wants lots of food at every meal. Somehow he or she doesn't feel complete unless the stomach is stuffed with food. The big-meal person can sometimes consume up to six fistfuls of food at every main meal. The big-meal eater usually prefers bulk to quality. This person likes supersize meals and thinks that all-you-can-eat buffets are a great value. Big-meal eaters think that a hunger pang is the cue to "order big and eat big."

The Binge Eater

Every couple of days or weeks, this person binges on food, any kind of food. Of course, binge eaters often have favorite food indulgences, foods that they have grown accustomed to binging on. Usually the binge eater eats to excess when alone, but you might find this person stuffing in food at a cocktail party or social event.

Thinspiration

The binge eater often uses eating to compensate for other problems in life. It is helpful either to address those problems directly by using self-help techniques such as journaling or by working with a professional counselor, or find a suitable substitute, like knitting or exercising.

The binge eater seems to go on automatic pilot and almost unconsciously (usually at night) eats and eats and eats until just below the burst point. He or she doesn't burst, but the body's sensitive and gentle communication system gets abused. A large amount of food makes the digestive system work extra hard. It not only has to digest all that food; it has to store it as fat.

Take heart. If any of these describe your habits, remember that you are not alone, nor "incurable." As you learn to listen to and honor your body's hunger communications, you will eliminate the unproductive habits that hurt your quest to reach your ideal size.

Developing a Hunger Scale You Can Use

Using a personal *hunger scale* is so fundamental to weight management that you will wonder why you didn't devise one long ago. Here's how a hunger scale works.

Lean Lingo

A **hunger scale** is a numeric system designed to help you "score" the hunger levels of your stomach at any time.

A hunger scale is any numerical system that helps you calculate the degrees of hunger and fullness you experience. The lower numbers on the scale represent physical feelings real hunger pangs; the higher numbers represent feelings of fullness that are uncomfortable or even painful (in other words, really *stuffed!*).

Our hunger scale measures hunger from 0 to 10. Here are the key reference numbers to understand:

Hunger Number	What It Means
0	*Empty:* The hunger point at which an infant cries or an adult has a hunger pang
5	*Satisfied or comfortable:* When an infant stops feeding or when an adult feels a neutral feeling, neither hungry nor full
7	*Full:* When you feel pressure inside the stomach from overeating
10	*Stuffed:* When you feel as if you are can't-eat-another-bite stuffed and are highly uncomfortable from eating way too much food

What's Your Number?

On a scale of 0 to 10—with 0 being empty, 5 being comfortable, 7 being full, and 10 being stuffed, what is your hunger number right now? Close your eyes and focus your attention on your stomach, which is somewhere around your navel. Set aside any analytical or intellectual data you have about when you last ate and simply let your stomach give you a number. By the way, when you hear its number, thank your stomach for the information.

What does your number mean? If it's 0, it is the ideal time to eat. If it is above 0, wait until your stomach registers 0 before you eat.

Toward the end of a meal—and definitely before you have second helpings—stop and ask your stomach what its hunger number is. If it's 5, stop eating. If it's 4, you have room for some more food. If it's 6 or above, stop eating and forgive yourself for having overeaten. Wait until you are at 0 before you eat again.

It's possible to get below 0. This can happen if you ignore your hunger signals, skip meals, have low blood sugar, or cannot eat when you are hungry. You could feel lightheaded, jittery, irritable, or headachy. The urge at that time is to "eat everything now." Don't do that. Instead, here is what to do if you get below 0:

Thinspiration

Using a hunger scale will give you excellent feedback about your eating habits. It can have a profound impact on your weight-loss efforts almost immediately.

◆ Eat a little something to get up to 0. This could be a piece of fruit, a cracker, juice, or some other food.

◆ Wait 10 to 15 minutes until your stomach hunger level is at 0.

◆ Eat normally, up to or below 5.

The beauty of this system is its simplicity. After you try this a handful of times, you will be amazed at the insights into your eating habits that you will gain.

Snacking the Right Way

Let's say you are planning to eat dinner at 7 P.M., but its only 5 P.M. now and you are already empty and feeling a hunger pang. You are at 0. This is a great time for a snack. You can eat a little something to get your hunger number up to 2 or 3 to tide you over until dinnertime. It wouldn't make much sense to eat up to 5 because then you wouldn't be hungry when dinner is served.

Snacks are great for whenever you are at 0 but it isn't mealtime. We can take snacks with us just in case we get to 0 when no one else with us is hungry. That way, we don't get overly hungry and famished. Overly hungry means you could eat the proverbial house. A little snack here and there prevents inhaling our food at the next meal.

Only eat snacks when you need them, that is when you are at 0 and it isn't time for a regular meal. Some people need snacks daily, some don't. Don't make of habit of having snacks just to have them.

Winning the Numbers Game

Are you superhuman? No. So don't expect to stay within the 0 to 5 hunger number range when you are first starting to use the hunger scale. Old habits die hard. Please don't beat up on yourself mentally when you overeat. It is terribly counterproductive. Forgive yourself, but determine to listen to your body better the next time you eat. And the next time. The more often you eat to 5 or less, the quicker you will reach your ideal size.

The following table is a simple guide to help you record your hunger numbers both before and after eating for a week. Eventually, you will keep track of your hunger numbers without writing them down. They will become second nature to you, and eating by the numbers is one of those "good eating habits" you will develop and rely on.

Your Hunger Number Chart

Day	Mon	Tues	Weds	Thurs	Fri	Sat	Sun
Breakfast beginning							
ending							
Snack beginning							
ending							
Lunch beginning							
ending							
Snack beginning							
ending							
Dinner beginning							
ending							
Snack beginning							
ending							

The Least You Need to Know

- Your body instinctively knows when to eat and when to stop eating.
- Only eat when your stomach is hungry.
- Stop eating when you have had enough food but before you are full.
- The size of your stomach is about the size of your fist.
- By using the hunger scale from 0 to 10 and only eating from 0 to 5, you are using a convenient approach to listen to your body's hunger signals.
- Snacks are a great way to honor your body's hunger signals.

Starve Your Body, Gain Weight

In This Chapter

◆ How a caveman's biology affects your weight loss

◆ Avoiding starvation metabolism

◆ Taking advantage of your powerful biological eating force

◆ Boosting your metabolism

Have you ever wondered why you gained your weight back after successfully losing it? You don't lack willpower or self-discipline. Instead, you are the victim of your own biology. Your biology makes you regain weight just as fast as you took it off. To keep weight off, you need to learn how your biology works and how to work with it to get to your ideal size and stay there.

You will learn how many of the popular diet recommendations can actually make you gain weight in the long term and make it harder to lose weight after that. You will learn how to avoid yo-yo dieting and the flabbier body that goes with it.

The Caveman and You

Your body is utterly amazing. From the food it consumes, it derives energy and nutrients. What your body doesn't need for energy, it stores as fat for later use.

The good news is that your stores of fat are great protection against an upcoming famine. Like most mammals, humans with a good layer of fat on their bodies can live for several weeks without eating. You may get restless when you haven't eaten in a few hours, but the truth is that you could live quite a while before your next meal. You would eventually feel weak and lethargic, but you could still survive.

So hooray for fat, your protection against famine! But what happens when that famine never comes? As long as you keep eating more than your body needs for fuel, the body keeps storing more fat. Today in the United States, most of us don't need to concern ourselves with fear of not having enough food, but our biology is still quite primitive. It is very close to that of our ancient ancestors, the caveman and cavewoman. Our present-day genome, the basic human genetic code, is almost identical to humans who lived 40,000 years ago. Yes, we rely on cell phones and computers, automobiles and airplanes, but biologically we aren't much different from humans who lived during the Stone Age.

The caveman lived between the extremes of feast and famine. When he was fortunate enough to kill a large mammal, his whole family—perhaps even the whole tribe—feasted on the delicious meat. It provided high-quality protein, fats, B vitamins, and trace minerals that the caveman needed for survival. Meat provided these in bioaccessible concentrations better than any other single food source. At other times, the lean times, the caveman ate berries, fish, and plants to get by until he once again killed more game.

Lean Lingo

The general term **metabolism** refers to all the changes occurring in digested foodstuffs in the body from their absorption until their elimination. Your basal metabolism is the rate of energy metabolism required to keep the body alive. As you increase your metabolic rate, getting to your ideal size is easier.

During times of famine, the caveman's *metabolism* would slow down to conserve energy. When possible, his body would increase his fat stores by taking even the meager amounts of food he did eat and storing it as fat. Why fat? Because fat is a more efficient fuel than muscle. The more fat that was stored, the longer the caveman could survive during a famine.

When he and the other members of the tribe feasted on the game meat, they were enjoying excess and abundant food. The caveman's body was clever. It knew that there could be a famine in the future, so it planned for contingencies. Any excess eaten food was stored as fat to prepare for the famine to come. The body handled the natural swings of feast and famine in elegant ways that ensured the survival of the species.

Your biology is designed to do exactly what the caveman's did. Your body will conserve energy and store fat when it senses that it isn't getting enough food and nourishment, and your body stores fat when you overeat. Does this sound as if you are in a double bind? You add body fat if you undereat, and you add body fat if you overeat.

The solution to the dilemma is fundamentally simple: Get enough food on a day-to-day basis for energy and nutrition, but not more than enough and not less than enough.

Your Body Is an Engine

Your body acts like an engine that is constantly in operation. Food is its fuel. It burns the fuel to keep going. But your body's engine really consists of millions of living cells, which are themselves tiny engines. Each cell in your body requires energy to stay alive. Food provides the energy.

In Chapter 9, you will learn how the body derives the energy and nutrients it needs from foods. For now, however, think of your body as a marvelous engine that keeps you alive by converting food into energy through a number of chemical processes.

Your metabolic rate measures the rate at which your particular body is using up energy (as measured in *calories*) to stay alive. It is not a rate that remains constantly the same. Your metabolic rate varies throughout the day, depending on your level of activity and other factors.

Your basal metabolic rate (BMR) describes the rate at which your body uses energy (also measured in calories) in a totally relaxed mode. It is usually measured in the morning after a comfortable night's rest, when you are relaxed in bed, before breakfast. (Sounds nice, doesn't it?!)

Lean Lingo _____

A **calorie** of food refers to the amount of energy available to the body from the oxidation or digestion of food. In science, a calorie is technically defined as the amount of heat required to raise the temperature of one gram of water one degree centigrade. When used as a calorie of food, it means that when a food is oxidized in the tissues of the body, it releases 1,000 times that amount of energy to be used by the body.

A Closer Look at Metabolic Rate

John, a 28-year-old mechanic whose hobby is mountain biking, claims to have a "high metabolism." He probably believes that his basal metabolic rate is higher than the norm. He may be right. We don't all have the same BMR. The following are known to influence basal metabolic rate:

- **Age.** BMR gradually decreases with age due to inactivity and lower muscle mass.

- **Sex.** The rate is generally a little lower in women than in men.

- **Sleep.** Inadequate sleep over time will decrease BMR.

- **Exercise.** Systematic exercise will increase BMR.

- **Nourishment.** Prolonged undernourishment will decrease BMR.

- **Thyroid hormone.** Poor thyroid functioning decreases BMR.

John, because he's young, muscular, and athletic, probably does have a higher basal metabolic rate than Jim, a middle-aged accountant who struggles to push the lawn mower on Saturdays. John's higher BMR will help him burn calories faster than Jim does … even when he's asleep. His engine is idling faster; it uses up fuel faster.

But John may have been referring to the fact that he burns through a lot more calories every week because his overall metabolism operates at a higher level. The physical activities he engages in, both at work and in leisure, burn calories faster than sedentary activities. His engine is working harder; it uses up fuel even faster.

The rate at which you burn calories is lowest while you sleep and greatest when you physically work hard. Here's a guide that describes the approximate calories burned during various types of work. Keep in mind that these "burn rates" will vary from person to person, so use this as a guide to the relative energy used up for each level of activity.

Activity	Calories Per Hour
Sleeping	65
Very light work or sitting at rest	100
Light work	120
Moderate work	175
Heavy-duty work	375

As you can see, energy stored in the body is metabolized much more quickly when physical exertion increases. So let's compare the calories burned in a typical day by John and Jim.

John	Calories
8 hours of sleep at 65 cal/hr	520
8 hours of work as a mechanic at 175 cal/hr	1,400
4 hours of everyday light activity at 120 cal/hr	480
2 hours of mountain biking at 375 cal/hr	750
2 hours of eating, TV, etc. at 100 cal/hr	200
Subtotal	3,350
Calories burned during digestion (10%)	335
Total requirement for 24 hours	3,685

Jim	Calories
8 hours of sleep at 65 cal/hr	520
8 hours of work at desk job at 120 cal/hr	960
4 hours of everyday light activities at 120 cal/hr	480
4 hours of eating, TV, etc. at 100 cal/hr	400
Subtotal	2,360
Calories burned during digestion (8%)	189
Total requirement for 24 hours	2,549

Without even considering that John probably has a higher basal metabolic rate because of his regular physical activity, you can see the dramatic difference in caloric requirements because of the lifestyle differences between John and Jim. John can eat 1,100 more calories in a day than Jim without gaining weight. Keep these numbers in mind as we progress through the book.

Starvation Metabolism

Our ancestor, the caveman, faced daily hardships that meant he couldn't always count on his next meal. During lean eating times, his body automatically went into *starvation metabolism*. So can yours. This is not good.

It's a cruel joke that our bodies will kick into starvation metabolism at the most inopportune time. We're not starving. We're just trying to lose weight! Most people who slip into starvation metabolism do so when they go on a highly restricted diet for a

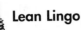

Lean Lingo

Starvation metabolism refers to a slowing of the basal metabolic rate brought on when the body is undernourished. The body, instinctively fearing starvation, naturally attempts to burn calories slower to survive longer. It also hoards energy, builds up fat stores, and causes the yo-yo dieting syndrome.

Weighty Warning

Going on a diet to lose just enough weight for a class reunion, wedding, or special party is ultimately fattening because your body shifts into starvation metabolism.

couple of weeks or a couple of months. Few people can sustain this kind of diet for long. Then, when the diet is abandoned, the dieter starts making up for lost time. The maintenance plan goes right out the door and in come the cookies, cakes, pastries, and candy. Adding insult to injury, the body then swings into excess mode and starts storing fat in anticipation of another perceived famine. Unfortunately, we willingly prolong the vicious cycle by again starting a highly restrictive diet.

The solution to this modern form of feast or famine is to eat balanced foods and nutrition in a weight-loss system that includes exercise, good eating habits, and positive thin thoughts. The system needs to be gentle, forgiving, and healthy so that a person can stay on the system over a lifetime, not just for a quickie weight loss.

Suppose you have already given up restrictive diets and have sworn off the ensuing compensatory food flings. You could still be putting yourself into starvation metabolism, perhaps on a day-to-day basis. Here's how you could be doing this and the corrections to make.

When you get a hunger signal from your stomach that you are now at 0 and it is time to eat, be sure you eat within an hour or so. Do not skip this meal. If you do, your body will get the message that food is not available and that it must start hoarding energy. It begins to store fat. If it's time to eat and you are not hungry—that is, if your stomach is not at 0—you can miss a meal and not go into starvation metabolism. If you are hungry, however, be sure to eat.

Monday morning is often diet morning. Sally, who repeatedly struggles with her weight issue, decides that this Monday is the perfect time to start a new diet. So how does she begin? She skips breakfast. Think of all the calories saved right off the bat. She also limits herself to some kind of light food for lunch, maybe even skips that meal, too. Sally is feeling quite proud of her willpower and self-discipline.

But come late afternoon when Sally arrives home from work, something inside her cannot stand it any longer. She might feel depressed, fatigued, and/or discouraged. She starts to eat and by bedtime has eaten enough food for three or four meals, getting more food than she needs. Overall she ate more food for the day than she eats normally. By evening, she was feasting. What happened?

By skipping a good breakfast and lunch, Sally put herself into starvation metabolism. The body started storing fat and slowed metabolism to conserve energy. By late in the day, Sally was "starving", so to speak, and her biology insisted that she eat. And eat our dieter did … to make up for the skipped meals. Within one day's time, the body had slowed metabolism, begun storing fat because the dieter was acting like she was in a famine, and later stored fat because the dieter was feasting.

For many people, the same scenario plays itself out day after day, and they are at a loss for why they are gaining weight. Even if dieters eat the same amount of calories in a day of feast and famine as they do on a normal day when they eat three meals plus snacks, feast-and-famine eating makes them gain weight.

The very best way to avoid slipping into starvation metabolism is to eat when your body is hungry. Skip meals only if your hunger level, as measured on the 0-to-10 scale, is above 0 (that is, it's 1, 2, 3, or higher).

> **CAUTION**
>
> **Weighty Warning**
>
> Sixty percent of women surveyed said they compensate for eating big meals by skipping meals. They put themselves into starvation mode. This is very fattening behavior. You won't be eating those big meals when you eat 0 to 5. Eating a big meal implies that a person ate way above 5, to full or even to stuffed, 10.

Eat for Optimum Energy and Metabolism

Your body likes balanced meals. When you favor one kind of nutrient over another, the body's metabolism can slow down. Judy was a 48-year-old woman who worked out at the gym doing cardio and weight training five to six mornings a week for at least 45 minutes. She was gaining weight. She insisted that she was not overeating.

We tested her metabolic rate and found that her metabolism was very slow and sluggish. She was confused. Wasn't the exercise supposed to boost her metabolism? What was happening to her?

We reviewed her eating over the previous couple of days. She had eaten no fat, no meat, and only soy shakes for meals. Her food intake had been like this for months. She wasn't getting enough calories, and her diet was out of balance. She was in starvation metabolism. Without enough fat and high-quality protein, the body acts like it is starving. Judy needed to add to her diet some essential fatty acids; perhaps some complete, high-quality protein such as meat, eggs, or real cheese; and plenty more vegetables and fruits. Only then did her exercise regime jump-start her metabolism and let her lose weight.

If you are not eating enough proteins, fats, or fruits and vegetables and are instead filling up on breads and starches, you could be in starvation metabolism. If you are centering meals around pasta and starches such as bread, wheat, rice, white potatoes, and corn, you could also be compromising your metabolic rate.

Gimme a Cup o' Joe

Oh, how we love our coffee and other caffeine-laden drinks! Unfortunately, they can be the enticing culprits that lead you into starvation metabolism. Let's say you have that first cup of coffee in the morning just after you awaken. It gives you zip and energy. It wakes you up. So far, so good. It can also keep you from getting hungry for breakfast. Not so good.

> ### Body of Knowledge
>
> Be sure to check the label on your favorite soft drinks and pain medications. Caffeine is contained in most dark-colored sodas such as Coke and Pepsi and is also in Mountain Dew.

Caffeine inhibits your ability to feel hunger. In other words, it gives you a false negative for hunger. So you most likely skip breakfast. Come midmorning, you want a little something to eat because your blood sugar has crashed. This is due to not eating and also because of the lift and drop caused by caffeine. If food is inconvenient at the moment, you may just settle on another caffeinated beverage.

You may actually be using caffeine as a way to not have to eat. Well, it works for that, but you are getting into starvation metabolism because you aren't eating regularly.

Recent studies have shown that drinking two to three cups of coffee per day can elevate cortisol levels. Cortisol is an adrenal hormone that adds weight around the waist and tummy.

Caffeine is in coffee and tea. It is an ingredient in many soft drinks and diet soft drinks, appetite suppressants, and over-the-counter painkillers, diet pills, and supplements. Caffeine is also in kola nut, guarana, and green tea.

> ### Thinspiration
>
> Breakfast is such an important meal that we encourage you to eat it even if you're not feeling hungry. This is the only time we recommend that you break the rule to eat 0 to 5. You need to become accustomed to eating a balanced breakfast with protein, fat, and carbohydrates. Eating breakfast revs up your metabolism for the day. After a while, you will become hungry for breakfast and your metabolism will benefit.

We know you love your coffee and caffeine, and the good news is that you most likely do not need to give it up. But you may need to change the way you use it. Rather than having your coffee or caffeine before a meal, have it with your meal and have only a cup or two in your day. That's right, have your cup of joe *with* breakfast, not before breakfast. The same goes for any caffeine you have throughout the day. That way, you avoid starvation metabolism and can still enjoy a cup of joe.

Boosting Your Metabolism

You've probably heard that it's important to keep your metabolism high to lose weight. You don't have to be content with a slow metabolism. Wishing and hoping won't enhance your metabolic rate, but doing the right things will. Here are effective ways to boost your metabolism and keep it high throughout your life:

◆ Make sure you do not inadvertently put yourself into starvation metabolism. If you do, correct the situation as soon as you can.

◆ Avoid overeating because this stalls the efficient burning of fuel. Eat from 0 to 5. Overeating forces the body to store more fat, increasing your body fat percentage. This slows your metabolism.

◆ Increase the muscle percentage in your body and decrease your body fat percentage. The higher the muscle mass, the faster you burn fuel. As you increase muscle mass, your basal metabolic rate increases. See Part 4 for information on how to exercise to increase lean muscle mass. You'll love how your body looks with more muscle and less body fat.

◆ Don't severely limit your intake of proteins, fats, or carbohydrates. Eat balanced meals so that your body has enough nutrition to keep your metabolism high.

◆ Get your personal ideal amount of sleep every night. Not getting enough sleep slows your metabolism.

> **Body of Knowledge**
>
> An equivalent weight of muscle is one third the size of fat. As you increase muscle mass percentage, you will be smaller and fit into those jeans.

◆ Use the power of your mind to propel yourself to a higher metabolic rate. Tell yourself that you have a high metabolism. Also be sure to keep saying aloud to yourself that you are at your ideal size. You'll learn more about this in Part 6.

◆ Avoid continually running on adrenaline or living with a chronic stress situation.

◆ Breathe deeply. Get plenty of oxygen. For fuel to burn, it needs lots of oxygen. Get this from exercise and from taking deep breaths that you can feel all the way into your stomach. This is called diaphragm breathing.

◆ Don't skip meals. When you're hungry, eat 0 to 5.

Body of Knowledge

When a person stops smoking, the brain acts as if it is low in the neurotransmitter serotonin and a person starts craving starches, such as breads and cookies. Nicotine acts as an appetite suppressant and it raises the metabolism to burn about an additional 100 calories per day. When a person stops smoking, they need 700 calories less per week than before, but they have the cravings for more starches. This easily makes for weight gain. Never try to quit smoking and lose weight at the same time. If you are quitting, be sure to use the stress reducers discussed in Chapter 8 to increase serotonin without eating the extra starches.

- Consider alcohol to be a food and factor it into your overall food consumption.

- Avoid watching TV or playing video or computer games for more than a couple hours at a time. When you watch television, your body's metabolism drops almost to sleeping levels. When we sleep, our metabolic rate is the lowest of the day.

- Just as you should only eat when you are hungry, only sip on sweet-tasting liquids when you are hungry, or at 0 on the hunger scale. Consider everything you put into your mouth, with the exception of water, to be a food.

- Drink plenty of water—at least eight glasses a day. Being hydrated increases your metabolism. More on your need for water in Chapter 13.

These guidelines will be used throughout the rest of this book as we discuss foods, exercise, and popular diet plans. We strongly encourage you to use these criteria to help you develop your weight-loss program. If your weight-loss plan violates these guidelines, you won't get the results you desire.

The Least You Need to Know

- If your eating habits swing between deprivation and excess, your body goes into starvation metabolism and stores fat.

- Your metabolism and basal metabolic rate are influenced by your lifestyle decisions.

- In starvation metabolism, your body instinctively hoards fat out of fear that it will eventually face deprivation or famine, and this slows your metabolism way down.

- You can avoid starvation metabolism by eating when you are hungry. On the hunger scale, eat when your stomach is at 0 and stop when you are at 5 or below.

- Balanced-eating food plans let you avoid starvation metabolism.

- Limit your intake of caffeine to meals only.

Chapter 7

Making Friends with Food and Eating

In This Chapter

◆ Learn eating behaviors that make you thin

◆ Mealtime is for relaxation and enjoyment

◆ Learn to eat beautifully

◆ Here's to your good digestion

Having a weight issue typically means having a love-hate affair with food. You may love to eat but hate what food does to your body and self-esteem. This love-hate affair can make your mealtimes challenging. You just can't seem to approach food in a simple, satisfying way. You're not alone.

In this chapter, we'll reveal how to turn your relationship with food into a love-love affair. We'll explore how to get the most out of every delicious bite while at the same time eating so that your body benefits the most from your food. Food will become your friend … *not* your enemy and *not* an object of unbridled desire!

The Pleasure of Food

Eating is truly one of life's most pleasurable and sensuous activities. Quite simply, food tastes good. It pleases all your senses of taste. Food offers delightful aromas and textures. It refreshes us. Enjoying food, especially delicious food, is one of the most natural experiences in the world. Hooray!

So why do we persist in our love-hate relationship with food? It's so unnecessary. Food in and of itself cannot make you fat. It has no such power. The power resides in you and your eating habits. If you overeat any food, you can gain weight. If you eat food using the 0-to-5 approach described in Chapter 5, you can get to your ideal size. In other words, food doesn't have power over you; you have power over food.

A Healthy Appetite Really Is Healthy

Just as hunger is a valuable feeling you do not want to avoid, so, too, is a normal appetite a good thing. Appetite is the desire for food, often for favorite foods or certain types of food. Your normal appetite for certain foods fluctuates from day to day. You should honor your appetite. Don't ignore or resist its natural function. For instance, you may have an appetite for eggs and bacon for breakfast. You don't have to resist your appetite and eat only cereal. Go ahead and eat the eggs and bacon.

Crazy About Those Cravings

Unfortunately, there is such a thing as false appetite. A false appetite is basically an irrational craving. Your brain becomes self-programmed to desire something so strongly that it incites you to compulsive consumption. Your false appetites often will be for foods that can be harmful, such as allergic foods, lots of sugar, and highly processed refined starches such as breads, pasta, cookies, and cakes.

Mike, a college student, is allergic to wheat, corn, and milk products. They give him stomach cramps and frequent diarrhea. He can't resist eating certain wheat products, especially sandwich bread … even when it makes him sick. His craving for bread can be so extreme that he will even put sirloin steak with cheese between two pieces of bread. Like someone who needs a daily fix of coffee, his desire for bread practically compels him to act irrationally. His eating habits are ruining his fun and activity. Of course, he can ultimately control his urge for these allergic foods by substituting other foods he loves that aren't harmful.

You can manage your appetite by directing it toward good-for-you foods such as the basics—meat, fruits, vegetables, and fats. If one day you have an urge for broccoli, give in to it. Ditto for steak, salmon, salad, and so on. Your body will be glad you did. You don't need to battle your appetite. Just manage it as one part of your overall eating approach. Part 3 of this book addresses in detail what you can eat.

Good Digestion Comes with Pleasurable Eating

Many people who are overweight have poor digestion. For the most part, poor digestion is not inherited or genetic. We give it to ourselves through the way we eat. Eating to soothe stress or anxiety is often the culprit.

Alas, poor digestion can lead to weight problems. Here's how: When a person feels stressed, the part of the central nervous system that regulates digestion switches off. This is called the parasympathetic nervous system. At those times of stress, the body can take in food and process some of it, but digestion doesn't work correctly to extract all the nutritional goodness from the food.

Poor digestion is not always obvious by observing symptoms. You could get heartburn, diarrhea, or constipation but not always. Poor digestion can be seemingly silent.

> **Weighty Warning**
>
> Poor digestion can lead to being overweight and obese. Improve your digestion by eating when relaxed.

If you eat when you are stressed, anxious, or nervous, you might as well be eating cardboard for all the nutrients your body gets. Yes, eating when stressed is a gaining situation. Now you might think, well, gosh, if I'm not digesting, the calories aren't getting handled, so I should be losing weight. Good idea but wrong reality. When digestion is impaired, the body starts "starving" from lack of necessary nutrients. Yes, it goes into starvation metabolism and starts hoarding fat and energy. It thinks it's in a famine. The good news is that it's easy to make some corrections and get rid of stress at mealtimes.

If you feel stressed often, it can be helpful to take a supplement of the multiple B vitamins. These help, but you could still find yourself stressed at mealtimes. Here's how to make meals a losing experience.

Eating with Elegance and Grace

Whether you're eating hamburgers on the patio, a hot dog at a baseball game, or a five-course dinner on Valentine's Day, you can use the following principles of eating with elegance and grace. Yes, even if you are eating with babies and small children, you can improve your digestion and enjoy your meal.

Eat Beautifully

Think back to your eating environments for the past three or four days. Have you eaten in the car, in front of the TV, or with your e-mail as a companion? Have you eaten at your desk or during a difficult and emotional discussion? Have you been so upset that you took your dinner to bed with you? In each situation, you're missing an opportunity to eat beautifully and healthfully. Eating beautifully means eating in an environment that is peaceful, health giving, and enjoyable.

Let's start with the basics. Beautiful eating is eating while seated at a table with utensils, plates, and napkins, maybe even with placemats or a tablecloth. Even better, include flowers, candles, and perhaps a centerpiece.

Next think about the sounds you want to hear when you are enjoying your food. Do you want to hear the evening news, a TV sitcom, or an argument the children are waging? Or do you want lovely music and even better conversation? You will enjoy eating—and will eat more intelligently—if you turn off the TV and focus on your food and your eating companions. Stop reading and just enjoy your food. If the phone rings, you don't need to answer it. That's what voice messaging is for—to handle phone calls when you don't want to. The phone ringing is not a good enough reason to interrupt your enjoyment of your food. Food is such a wonderful thing in and of itself that it doesn't need diversion. In fact, it's so wonderful that it deserves your full attention.

In a study of women, some ate while watching an interesting suspense story on television. The others simply ate their food without outside stimulation. The second group ate less food at the meal than those who watched the show.

Weighty Warning

One of our clients got distressed whenever she didn't receive a scheduled phone call from her boyfriend. Her solution was to order a pizza and take it to bed. Eating to soothe emotions while lying in bed is fattening and not beautiful.

The most fattening eating can be done when standing up or lying down. How many of us have shoveled in lots of food while standing in front of the kitchen sink staring out the window? Far too many of us. Eating while sitting sounds so fundamental. People who are at their ideal size are not the people who hover over the hors d'oeuvres at a cocktail buffet. They don't eat a full dinner while standing at the stove cooking dinner. Most adults who are at their ideal size enjoy beautiful meals. So whenever you are hungry, sit down and eat. Don't stand and stuff.

The best way to practice this principle of sitting to eat is to take all of your food and snacks to your place at the dining room or kitchen table. Eat your food there.

Eat Calmly

What have you brought with you to the meal? Set aside your concerns of the day when you sit down to eat. Believe us, they will be right where you left them when the meal is over. You can set guidelines for conversations at dinner. If someone insists on discussing things you don't want to hear about, you can put your fork down and wait until the person stops. You never need to eat even one mouthful of food in an environment or situation you don't like. Should your children act up, as children often do, you can also put your fork down until the ruckus abates. There's no reason to ruin good food by eating it in chaos.

You have the opportunity for three or more pleasurable eating interludes every day. Don't let them get messed up with less than pleasurable surroundings and activities. As best you can, eat beautifully at every meal. Yes, we know you can't always do this. But whenever you can and as often as you can, make your meals beautiful.

Slow Down and Lose Weight

By eating slowly, you give your stomach the best chance for good digestion. A meal should take a minimum of 15 minutes. Twenty minutes or longer is better yet. There are several reasons for this.

It takes about 15 minutes from the time when you begin eating for your stomach to signal the brain that it has had enough food and that it is satisfied and comfortable. Your mouth can consume food faster than your stomach can register that you have eaten it.

Thinspiration

Do you savor every mouthful of food you eat? Enjoying the taste of every bite is very helpful in limiting the quantity of food you consume. Eat slowly and be sure to chew each bite and swallow before you take the next bite.

If you eat quickly, you are more likely to overeat, easily reaching 6 or higher on the 0-to-10 scale. It is difficult to carefully and beautifully eat your food in less than 15 minutes.

Chew Sanely

We are often asked how many times a person should chew food before swallowing. Rather than answer this question directly—we don't want you to ruin your meal by counting chews—we prefer to think of it this way. Finish swallowing what is already in your mouth before you take the next bite. Before you swallow, chew thoroughly and try to chew slowly. Eating is not a race you win if you eat the fastest. Make every mouthful a delight.

Chewing is the first step in the digestive process. Saliva starts to break down the food and prepare it for the stomach. If you bypass chewing, your digestive efficiency is impaired.

The Least You Need to Know

- Make your eating a pleasurable experience; you will eat less food and be more satisfied.
- Ensure good digestion by eating only when you are relaxed and calm.
- Eat slowly and eat when seated, making sure to take at least 15 minutes per meal or snack.
- At mealtime, turn off the television and simply enjoy your food.

Chapter 8

Stress, Eating, and You

In This Chapter

- How stress can make you fat
- Mastering stress before it controls you
- The perils of eating when stressed
- Great ways to soothe stress

Losing unwanted weight will probably make you happier. Guess what? Staying happier will also help you lose weight! That's because ordinary day-to-day stress can inhibit your weight-loss program's effectiveness. That's probably no surprise to you. Stress affects us both physically and psychologically. For many of us, eating and stress are closely linked in a painful cycle that causes us to hold on to, or worse, add pounds.

Do the following situations sound familiar? It's a Friday night and you're feeling blue, so you munch your way through a bag of Oreos. Or you come home from work wound up like a ball of string and gobble a hefty piece of cake … before dinner! Or you sit down to lunch or dinner while taking care of paperwork and practically slurp down your meal without tasting it. You are doing stress eating. It's time to break the stress eating bad habits.

Running on Adrenaline Is Fattening

Living in a state of chronic and relentless stress actually adds pounds, regardless of what you are eating. You can have a very sound food plan and exercise regime, and your best intentions can get derailed because of stress.

Frank is a businessman who worked in a major city, but a few years ago he moved his family to a pastoral location 40 miles away. His morning and afternoon commutes were at least an hour long, even longer if there was snow or ice on the roads. By nature, Frank was a pretty high-intensity person, and the commutes made him even more tense and anxious. After a year, Frank's weight had increased 40 pounds, most of it around his middle. The commutes were ruining his dream of enjoying the countryside, so Frank and his family moved back to the city. His commute time dropped to about 15 to 20 minutes. Within six months, he lost the extra weight without altering his eating in any way.

During the long, congested, and sometimes treacherous commute, Frank's body instinctively shifted into fight-or-flight mode. Subconsciously, he was on ready alert and his *adrenaline* was working overtime. Even Stone Age men didn't have to run away from the woolly mammoth every single morning and evening five days a week for one to two hours! Yikes! While Frank's automobile ran on gas, he ran on adrenaline. He was under chronic stress.

Lean Lingo

Adrenaline is a hormone that directly affects the brain as a stimulus and indirectly affects our entire body. Our primitive ancestors relied on adrenaline for survival. Athletes today tap into their adrenaline to boost their performance. An adrenal hormone, cortisol, causes weight gain around the waist and midsection. To get rid of the "spare tire" waist, reduce the chronic stress in your life and get enough sleep.

When stress causes adrenaline to be excreted into the blood stream, along with it comes cortisol, a hormone that is responsible for putting on waistline weight. Recent research shows that when our bodies produce too much cortisol, we gain weight with or without eating changes.

Frank didn't move back to the city to lose weight; he just wanted more quality time with his family. He wanted more time … period. But a wonderful side benefit was that his weight returned to normal. By simply changing his home address, he consequently changed his weight.

If you can find a way to change your lifestyle to reduce stress significantly, do it. You will find that your weight issues improve or dissolve. Unfortunately, sometimes making the change is not feasible, as was the case with Laura.

Laura was an executive with a Fortune 100 company. Because of her work, most weeks she traveled from Sunday evening through Friday evening. Appointments were preset for her every day. She typically started her day with a breakfast meeting with one customer, called on customers all day long, and then ended the day with a customer dinner meeting. Her Friday dinner was often a not-exactly-gourmet meal on yet one more airplane flying home. On weekends, she did laundry, slept, and got ready for the next week.

> **Weighty Warning**
>
> When a person drinks beer and other alcoholic beverages, the body releases the hormone cortisol, which causes weight gain around the waist. They aren't called beer bellies for nothing!

Laura never enjoyed down time. She ran on adrenaline, not just three hours a day but virtually full time, day after day. She got by on just enough sleep, zonking out after finishing her business dinner and catching up on e-mails. She slept hard until the hotel wakeup call signaled that it was time to get ready for another customer breakfast. Laura was about 65 pounds overweight, and most of it was around her tummy. No weight-loss program had ever worked for her since she'd accepted her well-paying executive position.

Was it possible for Laura to slow the adrenaline rush? Absolutely. She could have exercised at the hotel's exercise facility before breakfast and enjoyed a warm bath every night before bed. By also being attentive to eating 0-5, Laura could have released her adrenaline-cortisol weight.

Running on Adrenaline Is Like Running on a Treadmill

So what good is cortisol? According to researchers, it probably served our primitive ancestors in a fundamental way. It helped them store fat. When we run on adrenaline, cortisol helps our bodies create new fat cells so that we'll have enough stored energy to give us a boost when needed. The bodies of both Frank and Laura got signals—completely unconsciously—from the adrenaline rushing through their blood to store fat … just in case the fat would be needed for a later energy boost.

Are you running on adrenaline too much? Work isn't the only culprit. Raising small children is often a fattening time in many women's lives. Although many women thrive in the milieu of motherhood, others get stressed out from the continual

Thinspiration

Relax fully every day to break the habit of running on adrenaline. Read a book, meditate, garden, stretch, or walk. Do positive, inspiring, and uplifting activities that are fun and that let you unwind.

demands of small children and household management. Despite the need to rush around, take care of everyone, and only snatch a bite to eat here and there, moms often still put on pounds! This just isn't fair.

You know if the stress in your life is too much. You know the intense feeling of an adrenaline high and the subsequent tumble into an energy low when the adrenaline stops. Look carefully at your life and figure out how to cut back on stress and adrenaline. You will likely be cutting back on your weight problem, too.

Stressed Spelled Backward Is Desserts

In times of anxiety, sadness, boredom, or nervousness, an overeater traipses off to the kitchen. The foods in the pantry or refrigerator seem to offer instant relief. She indulges her need for the pastries, cakes, cookies, crackers, and other yummy starches that will take away the bad feelings.

For someone with a weight issue, stress and eating usually go together like cream cheese on a bagel. They seem meant for each other. You wouldn't believe how many "confessions" we've heard about eating "an entire bag of cookies" or "a carton of ice cream" when feeling stressed!

Those who don't seek out food when stressed cannot understand this habit. They might listen to music, take a walk, or call a friend when they're out of sorts. But eat snack foods, "Why would I do that?" they ask. If you're a stress eater, however, you're probably right now shaking your head in disbelief that not everyone tries to eat away their blues.

Lean Lingo

Serotonin is a natural neurotransmitter in the brain that lifts mood. When we eat highly starchy foods such as cakes, cookies, bagels, and chips, more serotonin is released into the brain and we feel soothed.

Ever wonder why you don't gobble up steak and green beans at stressful moments? Because they don't work. They are just plain ordinary food. For most of us, steak and green beans don't have that magic something that elevates mood and temporarily anesthetizes the eater.

Starches like cookies, cakes, and crackers are definitely mood elevators. They increase *serotonin* levels in the brain, chemically altering mood and giving the eater a lift. In a sense, eating starches is not a bad choice when you are having a bad moment. Starches work. They make you feel better and are cheap. What's not to like? The answer: what they do to your body and self-esteem. They will make you gain weight when you overeat them.

Beating the Blues Without Feeding Your Face

Breaking the bad mood–munchies cycle is relatively easy once you find a great alternative to relieve stress. In surveying hundreds of overweight people about what works for them to soothe their anxieties and depression blues, we've come up with a list of excellent alternatives. The criteria for acceptance into our *Stress Soothers* Hall of Fame were demanding.

Stress soothers had to be all of the following:

- Legal

- Inexpensive

- Accessible (able to do at the office or simply by ducking into the nearest bathroom)

- Nonfattening

- Positive, inspiring, and uplifting

- Practical

- Realistic

- Quick

- Solitary (can be done by yourself)

Lean Lingo

Stress soothers are positive, inspiring, and uplifting alternatives to use when you're tempted to eat to soothe stress. The key to a good stress soother is that it redirects your interests away from the kitchen.

The suggestions that didn't make the Stress Soothers Hall of Fame were as follows:

- **Meditation.** It's a great idea, but it's not practical for most people at the moment of frantically needing to soothe stress.

- **Jogging.** This works great if you don't have small children at home, but jogging is typically not what a stress eater would do or would want to do.

Simple and Effective Stress Soothers

The activities that made the cut into the Stress Soothers Hall of Fame are the essence of simplicity and effectiveness. You are certain to find one or two of these that work for you during times of stress. They lift moods and can make you forget you ever considered a cookie fling just to make you feel better. You'll feel even better doing these!

Get in Water

Water works to lift moods. Take a bath, take a shower, get in the hot tub, or go swimming. Warm water envelops the largest organ of the body, the skin. It warms up every pore and relaxes the muscles.

When I (Lucy) was losing my weight over 20 years ago, I took baths long before I intellectually understood them. The most difficult overeating time of day for me was late afternoon. I found water to be the perfect relaxant. When I could get my hyperactive 3-year-old son to take a nap, I would hustle to the bathroom and enjoy a bubble bath. These were not necessarily long, luxurious baths; my son was likely to need me at any moment. Sometimes I took three-minute baths; sometimes they lasted for five minutes. But they worked.

I imagined that all the stress in me was going into the water and down the drain. By the time I put on fresh clothes, the urge to eat had subsided, and I looked forward to the rest of the day. Today, my grown-up son comments on how many baths I took when he was a baby. You bet, I say, they made me thin.

Get Warm

We are not bears. We don't need to add on a layer of fat to carry us through the winter, but some of us are inclined to act that way. When we are chilled, we are prone to eat more starches. You don't need to add pounds in winter to get more warmth. Wear clothes that are warmer and, when you feel chilled, put on your flannel PJs, get under the down comforter, and sip on a cup of warm herbal or decaffeinated tea. Getting warm can also divert the bad feelings.

Get in the Sunshine

Sunshine is the perfect mood lifter. Research indicates that 20 minutes of sunlight a day will naturally elevate your mood. Twenty minutes of sunshine daily also helps your hormones work correctly. People who live in the northernmost states or in areas of the country with lots of rainy days are often deficient in sunlight. The ensuing depression is called seasonal affective disorder (SAD). It can be remedied by exposure to plenty of natural sunlight or by using artificial full spectrum bright light, as provided by a *light box*. Sources for purchasing light boxes can be found in Appendix B.

Of course, it is best to get real sunshine. You can do this even if you work indoors. Eat lunch on the patio, take a walk during break time, or play outdoors with the children when you get home from work. Take a walk whenever you can.

Lean Lingo

A **light box** is a clever device that mimics natural full-spectrum sunlight. A small one stands about 16 inches wide and less than 2 feet high. It can sit on a desk or hang on a wall. Sitting in front of the box for even a half-hour a day can perk you up on winter or cloudy days.

Dry Brush Your Body

Purchase a natural-bristle brush or loofah from the drugstore or a discount store. It shouldn't be too stiff or too soft. With long strokes, dry brush your body. Start at your feet and work up your legs to your torso. Brush your tummy and buttocks. Then brush your arms, starting with your hands and working up to your shoulders. If you have a long-handled brush, brush your back. Finish up with brushing your chest and neck.

You will love this. It is so invigorating. It seems to make your body feel alive and refreshed. It can lift your mood. Dry brush your body before you shower in the morning or at any time of day when you feel a need to destress and renew your energy level.

Thinspiration

Although we recommend dry brushing your body for its mood-elevating effects, it also has some terrific health benefits. When you dry brush the body, you are assisting the lymph system in removing toxins. After a couple of weeks, you may notice that your skin is smoother and that even slight imperfections are gone. People who have done this for years report having skin like a baby.

Brush Your Hair

Doesn't brushing your hair sound almost too simple? Don't let its simplicity fool you. Across the board, clients who have tried this stress-soothing technique rave about its effectiveness. The best hairbrush for this technique is a very inexpensive one. Get the kind that has rough plastic bristles. The brushes with the fancy rounded tips don't work as well. We purchase ours at the big discount department stores.

Thinspiration _____

We love hair brushing to relieve stress because you can do it virtually any-where. Carry your hair-brush in your handbag or briefcase or keep it in the drawer in your office where you keep personal items.

To brush your hair, bend over from the waist and brush so that you can feel the bristles on your scalp. Brush enthusiastically for a minute or so and then stand up. Your scalp will tingle and will feel as if you are massaging your brain chemicals directly. We doubt this actually happens, but it sure feels that way. It's also great for your hair and scalp.

Just imagine, in just a couple of minutes of brushing, you could brush away the stress-induced urge to eat.

The Back Roller Rolls Away Your Stress

The back roller is wooden and looks like a rolling pin with waves in it. The waves correspond to your spine and to the erector muscles on either side of your spine.

Use the back roller to roll away your stress.

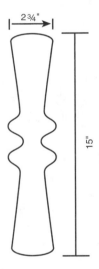

2¾"

15"

Lie face up with your spine in the middle dip of the roller. Beginning just below the neck, slowly move the roller from one vertebra to the next going down the spine. At each vertebra, breathe about 10 breaths and let your erector muscles on either side of the spine relax. It takes about 10 to 15 minutes to get all the way down the spine. By this time, you will probably be blissfully and totally relaxed. The urge to eat will have evaporated. When you stand up, your posture will be taller and you will be relaxed. Count on it.

Carry the back roller with you when you travel. It soothes the aches and pains caused by sitting on airplanes. Some aficionados love that it keeps their backs in alignment.

Others applaud how it stimulates acupressure points for all the major organs and glands of the body on its path down the spine. Others rave that it drains the lymph nodes on either side of the spine. Some claim it soothes their aching back.

You can purchase a back roller at some health-food stores and specialty stores that carry products for back care. It's inexpensive and lasts a lifetime. Information about purchasing a back roller can be found in Appendix B.

Having a Ball on a Ball

Body rolling is incomparable for deep relaxation. You can body roll at home and perhaps even in the office if you can shut your door during a break. For body rolling, you need an inflatable 6-inch ball. By simply resting your weight on the ball, the muscles close to the bone as well as the larger muscles relax. You can roll down the thighs and calves. You can roll up the spine and then roll up each side of the spine for a total of three times rolling up the back. You can include rolling up your abdomen. Use a smaller ball about the size of a tennis ball to roll on the soles of your feet.

It is best to have plenty of quiet time for body rolling so that you can experience deep relaxation over every nook and cranny of your body. We realize this isn't always possible. The good news is that you can still enjoy body rolling while watching the children or talking on the phone if need be.

Body rolling your whole body takes quite a lot of time, so you may want to pick and choose which body part to do at each session. You can produce great results in as little as one 15-minute session. We love body rolling first and foremost for relaxation. However, we have noticed improved posture and less cellulite. Where and how to purchase the ball with instructions can be found in Appendix B.

Sing Away Your Stress

As I was sharing the Stress Soothers Hall of Fame selections with my husband, he said, "Lucy, you forgot to tell them about the stones." I hadn't a clue what he was talking about. He said, "You know, the Stones. Every time the Rolling Stones come on the radio, your brain chemistry changes. You start dancing and singing along."

Thinspiration

Singing and listening to music have wonderful effects on your brain chemistry. Even if you can't carry a tune, it still lifts your spirit and lets you forget the day's stress and the urge to nibble away your anxiety.

It may not be the Rolling Stones for you, but everyone has certain music that makes him or her feel great. Maybe it's a favorite rock group from your youth or perhaps classical music you love. Maybe it's the Beatles, Beethoven, disco, or U2. Have these favorite tunes handy in your house and in your car, and when the bad feelings come that make you want to dive into starches, turn on your music and sing along. Just get in the groove of whatever music makes you happy.

So don't sing for your supper; instead, sing for your ideal size.

Hobbies and Games

Do you have a hobby, craft, or puzzle that you can pick up when you need to relax? Activities such as knitting, needlepoint, or crossword puzzles can so engage your hands and your mind that you cannot eat at the same time. A difficult solitaire game or a computer game may be all you need to get your energy headed in a new direction.

A half-hour or even 15 minutes of knitting can soothe and refresh you. Ditto a craft that you love. Whatever it is, however, you need to be able to pick it up right away and work on it. Find a hobby or craft that is readily accessible. Unfortunately, gardening is one hobby that you can't do as easily year round, but it's great during the planting and growing season.

Thinspiration

Think of your favorite stress soothers like you do favorite recipes. Write them out on a card that's posted in the kitchen, maybe right on the refrigerator. Use one of your stress soothers instead of trying to munch away your blues. They work.

Other possible activities in this category include reading magazines, polishing silver, art projects, journaling, and playing a musical instrument. If you've got a piano that is mostly gathering dust, tap on those ivories as a way to divert the blues. All of these activities will soothe the moods that otherwise might drive you to eat.

Long-Term Solutions to Short-Term Stress

The following activities may not work instantly, but over time they will help you reduce stress and the urge to consume serotonin-releasing starches.

Regular Massages

If you can afford massages, go for it. Even one massage every two to three weeks soothes ongoing daily stress. Massages ease tight muscles and can help the body detoxify through hand manipulation of the muscles and lymph nodes.

Stretch Away the Stress and Cravings

A regular program of stretching can reduce stress. Stretching releases the built-up tension in the body due to stress and anxiety. Stretch regularly, about three times a week. That way, you can release the stress held in muscles before it gets so big that you want to overeat to soothe yourself.

You can do stretching at home and in many semiprivate places. Many health clubs offer *yoga*, *Pilates*, and stretching classes. Stretching is recommended in most fitness programs, and excellent books and videos are available that cover stretching techniques. You will learn more about them in Part 4 of this book.

Lean Lingo

Yoga and **Pilates** are excellent forms of exercise for strengthening, stretching, and balance. Both techniques help you destress because they engage the mind as well as the body in doing the exercises correctly. Yoga originated in India many thousands of years ago, and Pilates was created by Joseph Pilates within the past 50 years. Pilates exercises create flexibility and overall strength to build long, lean, strong and fluid bodies. The exercises can seem familiar, such as a sit up or leg lift, but the execution is slower and more focused on posture and abdominal control than other exercise systems. More information about each approach is available in Part 4.

Aerobicize Away Your Stress

One significant benefit of aerobic exercise is often overlooked—*endorphin* release. By doing enough aerobic exercise, even as little as 20 minutes daily, your body releases endorphins that make you feel good all over and that override the feelings of bad moods and anxiety.

Take advantage of the natural system your body already has to improve your mood. Just 15 to 20 minutes a day of aerobics can lift your spirits for the entire day. You can also choose to do 45 minutes of aerobics three times a week. Find out which works best for you.

Lean Lingo

Endorphins are chemical agents released into the blood stream that stimulate the brain to feel good. Endorphins are released from several kinds of activities, including exercise, sex, and laughter. They are also released when we eat fatty foods, like chocolate and cheesecake, and starches, such as breads, cookies, and potatoes.

In addition to being good for your health, aerobic activity can chase away the cravings for the starches that lift serotonin levels. What a great bonus: Serotonin is a by-product of exercise that will help you control your eating! You will learn more about aerobic exercises that can work for you in Part 4.

Meditation, Contemplation, and Prayer

People in the throes of severe stress and low feelings often don't have the where-withal for meditation, contemplation, and prayer. We understand. However, these three spiritual activities can greatly assist you in staying in control of your moods and soothing your stress. When practiced often, preferably daily, spirituality can keep you focused on the big picture of your life. If any of these suit you, try them on a consistent basis. You will reap many rewards.

Stress Relievers You *Can* Consume

All of the activities that made the Stress Soothers Hall of Fame don't involve consuming anything. Here are a couple "consumables" that can reduce your stress level without adding weight:

- ◆ **Herbal teas.** Make sure these don't contain caffeine. Hot chamomile tea relaxes lots of folks, but you may prefer another flavor.
- ◆ **Water.** Preferably filtered, hot or cold. Drink it slowly.

An Overall View

You can use all of these remedies for stress when low moods send you to the refrigerator or cookie jar. Try them on for size and determine the ones that work best for you. Do one of the stress soothers before you head for the mood-altering starches. Stress soothers are great for you in many ways—for your health, your mental attitude, your relaxation, and best of all, attaining your ideal size.

The Least You Need to Know

- ◆ Chronic stress causes weight gain around the waist.
- ◆ Eliminate chronic stress by changing your circumstances if possible.
- ◆ Use techniques from the Stress Soother Hall of Fame to easily soothe short-term stress.
- ◆ To reduce stress in your life, take a proactive approach through daily activities that ease stress buildup.

Part

Using Food to Support Your Weight Loss

This part of the book is about food. After all, you've got to eat, and you won't get to your ideal size by *not* eating. In fact, eating well is essential to reaching your ideal size and staying there for life. However, you're much more likely to reach your ideal size if you understand how your body processes the things you ingest and then eat based on that knowledge.

Your body needs proteins, carbohydrates, fats, water, and other nutrients such as vitamins and minerals. In this part, you'll read straightforward explanations of the essential qualities of proteins, carbs, and fats and how to balance them in a safe, nutritious eating plan. You'll learn about essential vitamins and minerals and whether you should consider supplements or not. When you're finished, you'll come away with simple, practical guidelines that help you choose foods and prepare meals wisely … while attaining and maintaining your ideal size.

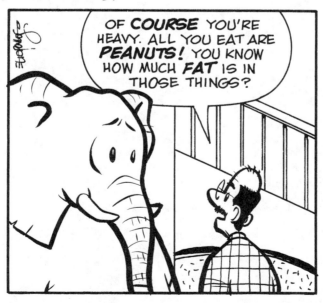

How Food Works

In This Chapter

- Fueling your weight-loss success with food
- Basic nutritional guidelines
- The new food pyramid
- Eating balanced meals
- Digestion essentials

Food, food, glorious food! By now you've figured out that we want you to be on good terms with food. Eating and getting to your ideal size really do go hand in hand. But what's a person to eat who wants to lose weight? After all, you've got to eat something. You've already heard enough—sometimes conflicting—advice to last a lifetime. So what should you eat?

You already know what *not* to eat. Certainly a Danish with coffee for breakfast won't get the nutritionist smiling. Neither will consuming a bagful of candy every evening while watching TV. Eating one donut is a treat, but eating a whole dozen is just plain dumb. A diet soda and a cookie for lunch is just asking for a weight problem. You recognize these no-no's. Now you just need to substitute the right foods into your overall diet. Your ideal size will be the reward.

Nutrition Counts

The science of *nutrition* gives us answers to this basic question: What do our bodies need? All the answers aren't fully known yet, but the study of nutrition has yielded valuable insights into how our bodies use food. By understanding some of the basics, you can make educated choices about your food intake and various diet and weight-loss programs.

Lean Lingo

Nutrition is the science that studies how various foods are required by the body for optimum health, which in turn helps you live at your ideal size.

To reach your ideal size, you will still need to eat. In fact, eating in certain ways will help you reach your goal. Isn't it wonderful that the very thing that made you overweight is also what will help you lose weight? You can't and don't need to abstain. So hurrah! You must—absolutely must—eat to get to your ideal size.

No Foods Are Evil

Unlike other experts you may have read, we don't believe in evil-food theories. No natural food is bad or evil, nor does it make you gain weight. So fat is not bad for you. Meat isn't either. Classifying foods as always good for you or always bad for you is disruptive to people who want to lose weight.

Thinspiration

Keep this important point in mind: All naturally thin people eat food, too, just like you do. You may be struggling with a weight issue, but your fundamental nutritional needs are the same as those of a thin person. You just need to learn new eating habits to reach your ideal size.

Chances are you've "learned" a lot about food as you've tried to deal with your weight. For example, you may know how many calories are in an orange and in a chocolate chip cookie. You can rattle off the number of fat grams in a pat of margarine or a serving of low-fat cottage cheese. You've been persuaded that some foods should be avoided altogether. Undoubtedly, some confusion may arise when one book says that a food is good for you while another book or expert pans that same food and applauds another.

Over the years, the list of bad-for-you foods has continued to grow. It's really getting silly. Here is just a small fraction of the foods that make someone's list of evil foods:

- Butter

- Red meat

- Chocolate

- Ice cream

- Cookies and cakes

- Sausage

- Cheese

- French fries

- Eggs

- Bananas (Yes, even bananas!)

You could probably add a dozen more foods that you've been told at one time or another to avoid.

We want to put the record straight. We are going to give you the up-to-date skinny on which foods are best for you, which ones are average, and which ones to eat infrequently. But we won't scare you. All of our recommendations are intended to both improve your health knowledge and understanding and assist you in losing weight.

The Forbidden Fruit Syndrome

You may find there are some foods you don't want to eat, but you shouldn't focus your efforts on so-called "bad" foods. When you believe a food is bad, you may give it the power of a forbidden food. Then something rather mysterious but really quite predictable happens—you want it more. You've turned it into the proverbial forbidden fruit ... only it's usually something more fattening than fruit!

People seem to love to eat what they perceive to be bad for them. If you talk with a hundred individuals who have weight issues, every one will tell you about his or her evil foods. It could be sugar or ice cream or donuts, perhaps potato chips or pasta. Yet they keep right on eating that food, perhaps even sneaking it so they can continue to get hidden pleasure because of its forbidden nature.

CAUTION   Weighty Warning _____

Perhaps you know that a certain food doesn't work well for you. Perhaps it makes you tired or gives you low blood sugar. In that case, it isn't the food itself that is evil; rather, it's your negative reaction to the food. Become attentive to how your body feels when eating certain foods so you can learn about the best foods for you and your body.

Here's how we recommend that you deal with your love-hate relationship with particular "evil foods":

Thinspiration

Make friends with foods that you thought were "evil" but ate anyway. You can eat all of your favorite foods as you lose weight but with less frequency and in smaller quantities than now. The secret is to savor your favorites slowly and in smaller amounts as you eat nutritionally balanced meals. Never overeat them.

Muster up your sense of humor and laugh at yourself! Then get over it. When you dispel your personal forbidden fruit syndrome, your counter-productive behavior tends to go away. If you can give up the illicit thrill of eating something you thought was bad for you, you'll disarm the power that food has over you.

The truth about all foods is this: Virtually any food can make you overweight, and any food can make you thin—it just depends on how you eat it. Remember to eat from 0 to 5 on the hunger scale. You won't go wrong.

Fill Your Tank with High-Octane Fuel

Food is your body's fuel. By now you have tried many different foods in your search for the fuel that makes your engine run optimally. If you want to manage your body so that it is a finely tuned, high-energy machine, you need to fuel it with high-octane food.

What makes good fuel for the body? We all differ somewhat from each other, and there's evidence that individuals from different ancestral backgrounds use food in their bodies differently. But you can count on a few rules of thumb about foods that fit into good high-energy diets. The best foods for you are …

♦ Part of a balanced diet.

♦ Not created in a laboratory. Seldom are the most nutritious and delicious foods designed in a corporate kitchen with lots of chemical additives. Rather, they are foods that humankind has been eating for centuries.

♦ Filled with fundamental nutrients such as vitamins and minerals that you need.

♦ Sources of energy that don't make you tired and instead give you sustained energy.

You know how you feel after a week or so on a highly restrictive diet. Not so great. Your body feels out of whack. You don't need to eat that way to get to your ideal size. The food choices we recommend will serve you well throughout your life. You won't need to relearn a new way of eating when you get to your ideal size. The same foods you eat to get thin are the foods you can eat to stay thin.

The Most You Can Eat

All the foods you eat need to be balanced and in good proportion with each other. Basically, there are three types of food plus a twenty-first-century addition. The three types of foods are as follows:

- **Protein.** The best and most complete sources of protein are meat, fish, seafood, eggs, cheese, and poultry. Other sources are nuts and legumes.

- **Fats.** These include vegetable oils (such as olive oil and sunflower oil), animal fats (such as butter), and fish oils.

- **Carbohydrates.** There's a vast variety of carbohydrates. They range from starches (such as breads, pasta, and rice) to sugars, fruits, and vegetables.

The twenty-first-century addition is …

- **Artificial foods.** We include this fourth type of food because it is prevalent in many of the items we buy at the grocery store. Artificial foods are usually designed in a test tube but are eaten either as a food or in food. Included in these are artificial sweeteners, preservatives, flavorings, and additives. These are found in many foods and are considered by the Food and Drug Administration to be safe for consumption. These are nonnutritive.

In Search of the Ideal Food Pyramid

In 1992, the government published recommended dietary guidelines to inform the public of the best and most nutritious way to eat. A basic concept in the guidelines was the food guide pyramid, which was designed to represent which foods you should eat the most of and which you should eat the least of. The food guide pyramid, taught in schools for decades and widely used by dietitians, was supposed to help you plan your overall diet.

At the top of the pyramid were fats, oils, and sweets. The next layer was dairy products and meats, including poultry, fish, eggs, and nuts. Below that were fruits and vegetables. The bottom foods were starches, breads, cereal, and grains. According to the pyramid, you were supposed to eat the most of these.

The long-standing food pyramid.

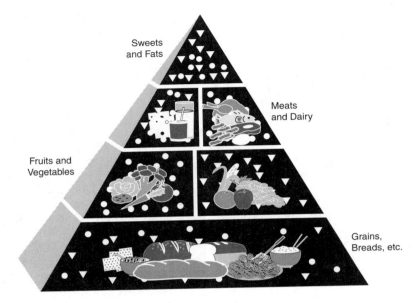

Old Food Pyramid

Revision of the Food Pyramid

Research that began in the late 1970s in Canada, Australia, and the United States suggested that this food pyramid needed to be updated. A new food pyramid was printed in the December 2000 *Women's Health Watch*, a publication of the Harvard University Medical School.

The fats and sweets are still on the top. You can eat some but not very many. The next layer down has grains, specifically low-glycemic ones. (Low-glycemic eating and the *glycemic index* will be further explained in Chapter 11 on carbohydrates.) Below that are meats, fish, and dairy products. Eat more of these than the grains. On the bottom layer are vegetables and fruits. Eat the most of these.

Notice the differences? The new food pyramid dramatically downplays the value of starches. Research indicates that eating lots of starches is putting our health and weight in jeopardy. Starches are indicated as a cause of high cholesterol, high triglycerides, and high blood sugar. In the new food pyramid, only one form of starch—low-glycemic grains such as barley and very-long-cooking steel-cut oats—is recommended. When eaten, low-glycemic grains create

Lean Lingo

The **glycemic index** is a measure of a food's capability to raise a person's blood-sugar levels. High-glycemic foods raise blood sugar a lot, low-glycemic foods just a bit. It's best for your weight and health to eat low-glycemic foods.

only a slight to moderate rise in blood-sugar levels. High-glycemic carbohydrates, such as potatoes, rice cakes, and white bread, create a quick spike in blood-sugar levels, which can contribute to obesity and a higher risk of diabetes.

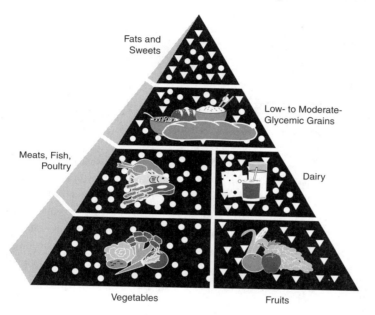

The updated-for-2002 food pyramid.

Suggested Food Pyramid

Also, the new food pyramid recommends that we eat five or more servings of fruits and vegetables every day. This is important. Eating lots of fruits and vegetables every day will enhance your weight-loss efforts—maybe dramatically. Consider all the good qualities of fruits and vegetables. They …

♦ Benefit your health with essential nutrients, vitamins, and *phytonutrients*.

♦ Provide fiber and bulk.

♦ Are available in many varieties.

♦ Can be prepared in innumerable ways.

♦ Satisfy your palate.

♦ Generally contain only a modest number of calories per ounce consumed.

Lean Lingo _____

Fresh fruits and vegetables are filled with **phytonutrients** that protect our health. They are the nutrients in plants that are beneficial to our health and well-being. Phytonutrients have been shown to help prevent such serious diseases as cancer, high blood pressure, and diabetes.

In making food recommendations, we will use the new food pyramid. It is more consistent with recent research and current thought on nutrition. The newest weight-loss programs are more geared to this approach.

What Is Bad Nutrition?

Here's a simple definition of bad nutrition: eating without consideration for your body's real needs. Too many donuts, too much coffee, too much protein, too much sugar, too many cookies, in essence, too much of any food isn't good nutrition. Ditto too little. If you don't eat enough fruits and vegetables, enough protein, and enough fat, you are also eating poorly.

Nancy was a typical American eater with 35 pounds to lose. Without thinking, she gravitated to high-glycemic starches such as breads and muffins for meals and snacks. She was much more likely to order a large sandwich for lunch than a salad or an entrée with a vegetable. At home, she would munch on chips and never consider eating fruit. Dinner often centered around some starchy food such as potatoes, pasta, or rice. Dessert was ice cream. At lunch and dinner, she typically drank a carbonated soft drink, one with either sugar or artificial sweetener.

Making the break from eating too many starches and sweets was a challenge for Nancy, but she persevered. She ate fruit with protein such as meat or cheese for breakfast. She took apples to work for snacks. She emptied her "emergency stash" of high-glycemic sweets that she kept in her office desk drawer and restocked with nuts, peanut butter, olives, and cheese and cracker snacks. She loved broccoli and made sure to keep some frozen broccoli in her refrigerator, and she learned to cook it several new ways for dinner. She learned to eat smaller, more varied lunches.

Nancy never completely gave up any food she liked—including ice cream—but she shifted the focus of her food selections. The ravenous hunger pangs decreased. Because of her new food choices, coupled with listening to her body's hunger signals and eating 0 to 5, the pounds started to come off. She felt better than ever and had more energy. As a result, she began an exercise program of walking and light weight training.

Avoiding bad nutrition is easy if you use common sense. Eating according to the new food pyramid will make you more successful on almost any weight-loss plan you choose. "Well balanced" needs to be your motto. Well-balanced means having some protein, fat, and carbohydrates at every meal and most snacks. Eating all foods in moderation is an ideal personal food policy.

Your Body as a Digestive Food Factory

Your body processes foods in much the same way that a factory uses raw materials to produce a finished product. The raw materials—the food you eat—go through a series of steps that convert them into muscles, fat, essential nutrients, and leftover waste products. Instead of picturing an assembly line, though, think of it as a disassembly line with your body taking the food in, breaking it down, and converting it into more useable parts. Fortunately, most of your body's digestive factory works without your direct involvement. Digestion is a highly complex process.

Good digestion means your food factory is operating smoothly. Poor digestion means some steps aren't working well, and the nutritional value of the foods you're eating is greatly diminished. Some people think that if they have poor digestion they will lose weight. It doesn't work that way. You can be both malnourished and overweight. The reverse is also true. You can be both well nourished and at your ideal size.

It's worth understanding some of the basic components of digestion … and what you can do to improve the process:

◆ **Chewing.** Your saliva starts the process of breaking down the food. Taking time to chew carefully gets your digestion off to a good start. Eat slowly so that you can thoroughly chew your food.

◆ **The stomach's excretion of adequate digestive enzymes.** These can be lacking due to genetics or aging. Some people do not excrete enough hydrochloric acid in the stomach to digest protein. Others do not naturally excrete lactase, which digests milk. If you have any indication that you do not have enough digestive enzymes, you can take a digestive enzyme supplement with each meal. See Chapter 13 for more information.

◆ **Relaxation.** The body digests best if you eat when you are relaxed. Be sure not to eat *to* relax; instead, eat only when you already are relaxed. You'd hate for all that good food to go to waste. If you eat when you're upset and nervous, you are essentially wasting food.

◆ **Absorption of B vitamins in the large intestine.** This process depends on you having plenty of the healthy *lactobacillus bacteria* thriving in the large intestine.

Lean Lingo

Lactobacillus bacteria is a bacteria that keeps the number of harmful bacteria in our digestive system in check. Without this, the risk increases for overgrowth of potentially harmful bacteria and yeast.

Stress has been shown to reduce Lactobacillus bacteria in our intestines. When this happens, the Bs don't get assimilated. B vitamins are our protection from chronic diseases, and they also aid us in managing stress. In fact, they are called the stress vitamins.

◆ **Elimination.** The fiber you eat in grains, fruits, and vegetables aids you in moving out waste products from the body. Your elimination needs to work regularly for you to lose weight. One client didn't go to the bathroom more than once every other week. To say the least, she wasn't eating enough fiber and her chronic constipation stalled her weight loss. Be sure you eliminate at least once a day. If not, first make sure you are eating five or more servings of fresh fruits and vegetables a day. If constipation persists, we recommend 25 to 30 grams of fiber a day plus plenty of water. Take one to two tablespoons of fiber daily. (An apple helps and so do prunes; whole flaxseeds also work well.)

Good digestion is essential for getting the full nutrition available from your food. In addition, good digestion reduces food cravings and lets you lose weight more easily.

The Least You Need to Know

◆ The new food pyramid is rapidly becoming the nutritional standard.

◆ All natural foods have their place in a nutritionally sound eating plan.

◆ Create good digestion to get the most nutritional benefit from the foods you eat.

◆ Give up classifying foods as good or bad and discover what foods work best for your body.

Chapter 10

Protein Means Power

In This Chapter

- The importance of protein for weight loss
- Getting satisfaction at mealtime
- Having plenty of energy to burn
- Practical mealtime suggestions

In our world of fast foods and convenience foods, eating high-quality protein can be hard to do. Yet without protein, your hair could fall out, your fingernails could crumble, and your muscles could deteriorate into, well, mush. Consuming enough protein is critical. You are unlikely to reach your ideal size—and stay energetic—without a steady diet of high-quality protein.

Think about it. In the right quantities, steak is really good for you! So are almost all lean meats, eggs, and cheeses. If you prefer a vegetarian diet, we show you how to get ample protein to reach your ideal size.

Proteins Are for Energy and a Whole Lot More

Proteins give you energy and are needed for your body to manufacture hormones, antibodies, enzymes, and tissues. Your body cannot live without certain essential *amino acids* found in protein. They're called "essential" because your body needs them to function properly, and it cannot manufacture them on its own.

You need a regular dose of essential amino acids in your diet. Yes, there are "nonessential" amino acids that your body needs, but it can synthesize them. (You'll learn more about this in the section that follows.)

When you eat a protein, your digestive system breaks it down into life-giving amino acids. As food travels through the gastrointestinal tract, your stomach and small intestine excrete enzymes that break the food down so that the nutrients can be absorbed into the bloodstream.

Your body uses protein as a raw material in the creation of numerous products that are critical for your health. After your digestive system converts the protein into amino acids, they flow through a large vein, called the portal vein, to the liver. The liver then passes the amino acids into the bloodstream, which distributes them to your tissues.

Your body's tissues, such as muscles and organs, select and store the amino acids they specifically need. These are used to synthesize new tissue or to maintain and repair existing tissue. Some of the amino acids are used to synthesize certain hormones and enzymes that are themselves critical to having your body function optimally and to letting you release fat stores. All of these processes are governed by the genetic intelligence encoded into each cell.

> **Lean Lingo**
>
> **Amino acids** are called the "building blocks of life." Protein from food is digested into amino acids. The amino acids are then used to build and maintain muscles and other tissues. They are also important in enzyme and hormone production.

> **Weighty Warning**
>
> Some individuals have difficulty digesting protein because their bodies aren't excreting sufficient enzymes (such as proteases and hydrochloric acid) needed for digestion. Clues that you may not be digesting protein well include soft, peeling, or splitting fingernails or a heavy, unpleasant feeling after eating protein. Certain dietary supplements, discussed in Chapter 13, can help you digest proteins.

The liver gets involved in the protein-digestion process in critical ways. It converts amino acids that aren't used by the tissues into other building blocks of the body. It synthesizes amino acids into fibrino-gen, the substance used in the blood to form a clot, purines, a class of protein that provides energy, creatine, an energy source for muscle contraction and many other chemical substances your body needs. The amino acids created from protein are also converted into energy.

Protein stimulates the pancreas to produce glucagon, a hormone that releases stored fat from your cells for energy. This process is necessary for weight loss. Unfortunately, the beneficial effect of glucagon can be blocked if you have excessive insulin in your bloodstream from eating too many starches and other high-glycemic carbohydrates. (See the next chapter for a full explanation.)

Protein strengthens your immune system and helps maintain the fluid balance in your body. Eating a meal that's high in carbohydrates boosts your metabolism by 4 percent. Eating a meal with high-quality lean protein boosts your metabolism by as much as 30 percent. Not eating enough protein can create digestive problems and fluid retention.

After water, protein makes up the largest portion of your body weight. This includes muscles, ligaments, tendons, organs, glands, nails, and hair. Protein is needed in your diet so that your body is healthy and functions properly.

Essential and Nonessential Amino Acids

The amino acids derived from dietary protein enable a host of things to happen in your body. For instance, the vitamins and minerals already in your body cannot be effective if the amino acids are not present. Two types of amino acids are considered to be biologically important to human life: essential and nonessential. The distinction can be confusing.

The essential amino acids are ones that must be obtained by consuming certain proteins. They're called "essential" because they can't be manufactured by the body itself. These amino acids are histidine, isoleucine, leucine, lysine, methionine, phenylalanine, threonine, tryptophan, and valine. Your body uses these individually and in combination synergistically to function properly. All of the other amino acids are nonessential, meaning that they are manufactured in the body; in fact, some are created from the aforementioned essential amino acids.

If you are deficient in some essential amino acids, it means your body doesn't have the basic raw materials it needs to function properly. You need to consume protein to obtain them. However, just because an amino acid is listed as nonessential doesn't mean your body doesn't need it. It only means that your body can manufacture that amino acid from the ones you've consumed. It is "not essential" that you eat it.

In the simplest of terms, all of this translates to one critical point: You need to eat protein. So how do you select which proteins to add to your eating plan?

Complete or Incomplete, Take Your Pick

Protein foods come in two versions:

◆ *Complete proteins* contain all the essential amino acids. These proteins are found in meats, fish, seafood, poultry, eggs, and cheese. These animal-based proteins

Lean Lingo

Complete proteins are foods that contain all the essential amino acids that the human body needs to build and repair muscle and body organs. **Incomplete proteins** contain only some of the essential amino acids, but they still offer significant nutritional value.

also contain high concentrations of B vitamins and trace elements that the body needs. Soybean products, such as tofu, tempeh, and soy powder, are not complete proteins because they lack methionine.

◆ *Incomplete proteins* contain only some of the essential amino acids. These proteins include grains, legumes, nuts, seeds, and some leafy vegetables. The yummy nut butters, such as peanut, almond, and cashew butter, are included among the incomplete proteins.

Combining Incomplete Proteins into Complete Proteins

Food combining is a good way to eat incomplete proteins. By eating certain incomplete proteins together, you can, in effect, get all of the essential amino acids at the same meal. To consume all the essential amino acids, you can combine legumes such as pinto beans, black beans, navy beans, and lentils with *any* of the following:

Lean Lingo

Food combining involves eating more than one kind of carbohydrate that contains incomplete proteins so that, when combined, you are consuming all the essential amino acids found in complete proteins such as meat and eggs. Recent research suggests that you don't have to eat the combined foods at the same meal, as long as you eat them within the same 24-hour period.

◆ Brown rice

◆ Corn

◆ Nuts

◆ Seeds

◆ Wheat

Or you could combine brown rice with *any* of these:

◆ Legumes

◆ Nuts

◆ Seeds

◆ Wheat

Traditionally, it was thought that combined foods needed to be eaten at the same time to get complete protein. New research suggests that people who prefer to eat vegetable proteins can make sure they eat the complete combinations over a 24-hour period, not necessarily at the same meal.

Every once in a while, most of us just gotta have a steak or hamburger. You know the feeling. You want something "meaty." Eating an entire loaf of bread or a giant salad just wouldn't hit the spot. Don't resist the urge; rather, give in and eat what your body is asking for. That inner craving can be your body's sensory language telling you that it needs some heavy-duty, high-quality protein.

Weight-Loss Benefits of Protein

By eating proteins at every meal, you provide yourself with enough nutritional support to keep going until the next meal. All the critical components for fat burning are provided by proteins. Without protein in our meals, we easily become tired. The most common tendency of people who don't eat enough protein for breakfast is to crash during mid- to late afternoon. They then overeat the quick, pick-me-up, high-glycemic starches and sugars. This is a sure way to gain rather than lose weight.

End the Late Afternoon Sags

Let's look at a typical woman who is trying to lose some weight. Faith starts her days with perhaps only a cup of coffee or some cereal and milk. Some days she eats granola and a carton of prepackaged yogurt. Then she skips lunch to meet a work deadline. Uh oh, trouble. By mid-afternoon, Faith starts dragging. It's an unpleasant feeling, especially because she really needs to tackle her work project. Almost without thinking, she seeks out food for energy. If a high-starch, high-glycemic snack (such as popcorn or a bagel) is handy, she quickly gobbles it down.

Faith's type of fatigue is common when someone doesn't keep stoking her metabolism with high-quality protein. You may be saying, "Well, what about the protein in that milk or yogurt? Doesn't that count for something?" Not much. A half-cup of milk has about 4 grams of protein. A half-cup of fruit-flavored yogurt has 4 grams. Neither has enough protein to give her zip into the afternoon. About 15 to 20 grams of high-quality protein at breakfast and lunch would sustain Faith through the afternoon and into the evening. Her late-afternoon, high-glycemic munchies would be tamed, and she would arrive home feeling energetic rather than famished and fatigued.

As for Faith's skimpy breakfast … the long and short of it is that with only 4 to 6 grams of protein, Faith hasn't stoked her engine with enough fuel to carry her through the day. By the way, even if she ate some protein for lunch, it wouldn't entirely make up for a deficient or nonexistent breakfast.

Your Basic Protein Requirements

The ideal amount of protein to eat on a daily basis ranges from 50 grams to 100 grams, based on the recommendations of various experts. Protein needs vary based on sex, body size, muscle mass, and activity level. So, doing some simple math here, you need about 16 to 33 grams of protein per meal, based on eating three meals a day. If you consume a protein snack, lower the grams of protein you eat at regular meals.

Different foods have different protein density. "Grams of protein" refers to the amount of available protein, not the weight of the food. For example, a 3-ounce hamburger has 22 grams of protein; a 4-ounce beef filet mignon has 36. Filet is the denser meat as far as protein goes.

> **Body of Knowledge**
>
> Depending on your normal activity level, you need 50 to 100 grams of protein a day for good nutrition. Women require less, men need more. On the average, there are 7 grams of protein per one ounce serving, so you need between 7 to 15 ounces of protein foods every day.

Obviously, some foods are more protein dense than others. One half-cup of cooked kidney beans has 7 grams of protein, one half-cup of chicken salad has 17, and one half-cup of cottage cheese contains 17. If counting grams isn't your thing—and we have to admit, it's not ours either—you can estimate by size. Figure that an average-size serving of complete protein needs to be about the size of a deck of playing cards. For incomplete proteins, such as legumes, you may need to double or triple that size to get the nutritional equivalent.

When you shop for meat and poultry, if possible, purchase organic brands or meat certified as grown without antibiotics or growth stimulants.

Use the following table to figure out which foods to eat. If you want more detailed information on all foods, you can purchase a protein counter at your bookstore or heath-food store. (See Appendix B for suggestions.)

Protein Grams in Food with Serving Size Suggestions

Food	Serving Size	Protein (Grams)
Almonds	¼ cup	7
Bacon	One slice	2
Baked beans	½ cup	8
Bean sprouts	½ cup	1
Beef, filet	4 oz.	36

Food	Serving Size	Protein (Grams)
Cheese	1 oz.	6–7
Chicken drumstick	One	12
Chicken livers	One	6
Chicken meat	3 1/2 oz.	32
Clams, raw	3 oz.	11
Cottage cheese	1/2 cup	17
Crab meat	1/2 cup	9
Egg	One large	7
Flounder	3 oz.	19
Haddock	3 oz.	21
Ham, boiled	2 oz.	14
Hamburger	3 oz.	22
Lamb chop	4 oz.	20
Liver, calf	2 oz.	15
Lobster	1 cup	20
Mackerel	3 oz.	20
Milk, skim	1/2 cup	4
Milk, whole	1/2 cup	4
Oysters, raw	1/2 cup	11
Peanut butter	2 tbsp.	8
Pork roast	3 oz.	19
Red snapper	3 oz.	22
Salmon	3 oz.	22
Shrimp	3 oz.	22
Soy Powder	1/3 cup	25
Soybeans, cooked	1/2 cup	14
Steak	3 oz.	24
Tofu	4 oz.	10
Tuna, canned	3 oz.	26
Turkey	3 1/2 oz.	31
Veal	3 oz.	23
Yogurt	1/2 cup	4

Low Blood Sugar Be Gone

Weighty Warning

Some low-blood-sugar situations for women are also associated with hormonal cycles. You may experience the effects of low blood sugar in the days prior to your menstrual period even when you eat balanced meals including protein, but they should become lulls and not crashes.

When you eat the recommended amount of protein at each meal, chronic low blood sugar can be a thing of your past and not of your new thin self. This is important. Far too many people get stuck in yo-yo eating, starving themselves one moment and then eating high-glycemic-loaded meals when their energy is gone.

You are way less likely to have your hunger numbers below 0 when you eat enough protein for breakfast, lunch, and dinner. That's not to say that eating protein completely solves low blood sugar. Proper eating of fats and carbohydrates will also help manage your energy level.

Ahh! I Feel So Complete After This Meal

By eating adequate protein, you will leave the table with a satisfied feeling of completeness, and it's a feeling that can last. You know the old joke about eating Chinese food—no matter how much you consume, you're hungry an hour later. You guessed it: Chinese foods contain very little protein plus the unnatural substance of MSG, which doesn't help. (This will be covered in Chapter 13, which discusses other types of consumables.)

Eating satisfaction comes from making all your senses happy. The aromas, tastes, and textures of protein foods just naturally appeal to both our prehistoric nature and our modern, sophisticated palates. Many people naturally eat less when they eat enough protein.

Protein! It's What's for Breakfast

You have heard over and over again that you need to eat a good breakfast to lose weight. We agree. Breakfasts that include protein are absolutely essential for keeping your energy high all day long and avoiding late-afternoon slumps. Protein elevates your metabolic rate throughout the day and night. It also helps keep you alert by stimulating the brain chemical *dopamine*. So plan on eating 15 to 20 grams of protein every morning.

That said, how do you do it? Getting adequate protein at breakfast is generally more challenging than getting enough for lunch and dinner. Why? The first reason is that people don't think of breakfast as a meat or fish meal, but think of those great breakfasts served in Great Britain! Fruits, meats, fish, cold cuts, eggs, and cheeses are all offered for a traditional "full English breakfast."

Second, preparing meat or fish for breakfast seems inconvenient. We understand. Many are the days when we wish there were a short order cook in the kitchen who could just whip up bacon and eggs for us every morning! Alas, we have to prepare breakfast for ourselves and our families. That's why we have compiled the following easy ways to get breakfast protein:

- Plain eggs
- Steak and eggs
- Egg omelet with cheese
- Huevos rancheros
- German pancakes, made with lots of milk and eggs
- Minute steaks
- Sliced ham
- Sausage or bacon (with as few additives as possible)
- Leftover meat from last night's dinner
- Chicken livers
- Barbeque pork
- Sliced turkey, ham, roast beef, and cheese (preferable to cold cuts like bologna and salami that can be full of nitrates and nitrites and high in sodium)
- Baked fish from the deli
- Tuna salad made with real mayo
- Salmon salad made with real mayo
- Chicken salad made with real mayo

Lean Lingo

Dopamine is a brain neurotransmitter. An increase in dopamine often leads to an improvement in mood, alertness, and sex drive, and perhaps an increase in verbal fluency and creativity.

Thinspiration

Cook your dinners so that you'll have breakfast leftovers. Some leftover roast beef, hamburger, ribs, cheese-and-chili casserole, turkey, or chicken, maybe alongside a scrambled egg, makes for a quick nutritious breakfast.

We will discuss why you should use real mayo in Chapter 12.

The following on-the-run proteins are for when you have to eat in your car on the way to work. Of course, we never recommend doing this, but we know what the real world is like. We live in it, too.

Weighty Warning

You may be asking why we haven't included soy shakes or protein bars among our breakfast suggestions. It's because neither are simple to recommend. Not all soy shakes or protein bars are created equal. We will tell you all you need to know about both in Chapter 14.

Breakfast proteins for eating in your car:

- Cheese
- Pre-peeled hard-boiled eggs
- Breakfast burrito with meat, beans, cheese, and so on
- Meat and cheese rollups
- Leftover meat, casseroles, stews
- Cheese and fruit

Our vegetarian friends tell us that they eat eggs, and/or cheese to get their complete proteins, which is terrific. You can also add some seafood like shrimp to your first meal of the day.

Protein Will Keep You Healthy

As we said, protein is your friend. It is literally the stuff that a beautiful body is made of—it makes for lovely hair, healthy nails, and the shapely curves or muscles you desire. Protein stimulates the fat-burning hormone glucagon, supplies the amino acids needed for new tissue, and helps elevate your resting metabolic rate (even when you're asleep!). Protein needs to be one of the mainstays of your diet. Eat it at least three times a day and preferably with every meal and snack.

The Least You Need to Know

- By eating adequate protein, your body obtains the building blocks of life, the essential amino acids.
- Complete proteins are found in meats, seafood, fish, poultry, eggs, and cheese; sources of incomplete proteins include soybeans, nuts, seeds, and grains.
- Protein gives you energy, staves off fatigue, and helps regulate blood sugar.
- If you eat protein for breakfast every day, you will love the energy it gives you.
- Protein helps you reach your ideal size.

Carbohydrates

In This Chapter

- ◆ Understanding how carbohydrates work
- ◆ Fulfilling your body's need for high-quality carbohydrates
- ◆ Eating carbohydrates to reduce fat stores
- ◆ The fab five a day—veggies and fruits

Carbohydrates are often the most poorly understood of foods. When many people talk about carbohydrates, they actually mean starches and sugars. Carbohydrates are the most varied of the three nutrient types. They include starches such as bread and potatoes, as well as sugars, fruits, vegetables, and of course, a common favorite, chocolate.

There's growing evidence (bad pun!) that Americans in particular consume vast quantities of fat-producing carbohydrates—and our waists are showing the results. Here's your chance to get a better understanding of how to eat carbs wisely.

Carbs Are for Energy

Almost all carbohydrates come to us from plants. The only animal products that contain carbohydrates are milk and milk products. Most people—and especially people who are overweight—love carbs, especially starchy cakes, cookies, pastas, and bagels. If this describes you, now is a great time to become acquainted with the full range of fabulous carbohydrates so you can more easily get to your ideal size.

Carbs come in two groupings: simple carbohydrates and complex carbohydrates. Simple carbohydrates are often called simple sugars. These include fructose (fruit sugars), sucrose (table sugar), and lactose (milk sugar). Complex carbohydrates are also made up of sugars, but their molecular structures contain longer and more complex chains of sugars. These carbohydrates include fibrous foods and starches. Foods high in complex carbohydrates include most green vegetables, whole grains, and beans.

Your body needs carbs for many reasons. They are the main source of blood glucose, the major fuel for all your cells and the only source of energy for both the brain and red blood cells. Yes, you do need to eat your carbs. Both simple and complex carbohydrates are converted into glucose in the small intestine. The glucose proceeds to the liver, your body's phenomenal processing system. The liver converts the glucose into glycogen, stores the glycogen, and subsequently converts it back to glucose as needed by the body's cells.

The liver also makes sure your bloodstream is getting only the glucose the body needs. So what happens to the excess glucose from an excess of carbohydrates? You guessed it. Your liver converts the excess glucose into fatty acids and stores it as body fat.

Your brain, with its many complex chemical reactions, gets a mild tranquilizing effect when you eat carbs. Carbs lift your serotonin levels. You have experienced this effect if you have ever used carbs to soothe anxiety, nerves, or a low emotional feeling.

Body of Knowledge

Many carbohydrates contain fiber. Generally, the less processed the food, the higher the fiber content. Fiber aids in digestion because it retains water and adds bulk, thus helping with proper elimination. High-fiber diets have been shown to help lower cholesterol levels because the fiber absorbs the fat in the body, thus lowering fat levels; and to reduce the incidence of colon cancer by absorbing toxins and moving them quickly through the digestive system and out of the body.

Carbohydrates Are Required for Good Health

Researchers are now discovering that some sugars are necessary for cell-to-cell communications and optimal immune response. As you might guess, these sugars aren't found in candy bars. Too bad!

The necessary saccharides are mannose, glucose, galactose, fucose, xylose, N-acetylglucosamine, N-acetylgalactosamine, and N-acetylneuraminic acid. Glucose is easy to add to your diet because almost all carbohydrates break down in the small intestine into monosaccharides such as glucose. The other necessary saccharides aren't as readily available in our modern diet. Fortunately, they are found in various vegetables and fruits, so eating a wide variety will help keep your health and immune system in order.

Carbs, Insulin, and Your Weight

Not all carbohydrates are created equal. Some definitely are better for you than others. That's because different carbohydrates affect blood-sugar levels differently. Some can really cause dramatic, unhealthy jumps in your blood sugar.

The glucose in our bloodstream is our primary source of energy. We simply can't live without a sufficient amount. But if there ever was a perfect example of "too much of a good thing," blood sugar is it. When you eat a carbohydrate, it lifts your blood sugar. This is when the pancreas goes into action. The pancreas secrets a hormone called *insulin*. Insulin works to keep your blood sugar stable so that you do not have sustained high blood sugar. This is the mechanism that doesn't work well for diabetics. So far, so good. You eat some carbs, your blood sugar rises, your pancreas secretes insulin, and your blood sugar level returns to normal. This happens every time you eat carbohydrates. This is normal.

Herein lies the rub. Some carbohydrates cause blood-sugar levels to jump higher than others. This causes the pancreas to excrete more insulin to stabilize your blood sugar. Because of the spike in blood sugar, the pancreas in a sense overreacts and puts out lots of insulin. After your blood sugar stabilizes, there can be extra insulin hanging around in your blood stream.

What are the consequences of excess insulin in your bloodstream? Insulin does what insulin is supposed to do:

Lean Lingo

Insulin is a hormone secreted by the pancreas gland. It regulates the level of sugar (glucose) in the blood. It's also one of the hormones that causes the body to store fat.

Body of Knowledge

If someone continually has high blood sugar, the body's cells become insensitive to insulin, and blood sugar can't leave the bloodstream. Someone with a fasting (meaning the person hasn't eaten for 12 to 14 hours) blood-sugar level of 120 or above probably has type 2 diabetes. Normal, healthy blood-sugar levels range between 75 and 115. The guidelines measure milligrams of glucose per one-tenth liter of blood.

1. **It makes you hungry again right away.** Think of when you start the day with a donut. Soon after eating it you feel hungry again, so you eat another one and then another one. Pretty soon the box is empty. Too much insulin in your blood stream can give you a sense of false hunger. Naturally, you want to avoid this.

2. **It stores fat.** Yes, excess insulin causes the body to increase body fat. This means you could be on a low-calorie diet and still be storing fat because of your choice of quick-acting carbohydrates. Ah-ha, you may be saying, that explains it!

Ideally, you should avoid eating quick-acting carbs and instead dine on the ones that do not trigger a fast insulin response. We have seen many, many overweight people finally begin to master their weight when they learn how to manage their carb intake. It's exciting.

The Carbohydrate Hit List

So what carbs are the "thinnest?" First in Australia, then in Canada, and finally in the United States, researchers have been educating the public about a concept called glycemic indexing. The index is a measure of the blood sugar response of various foods.

The research behind the glycemic index is simple and makes sense even to nonscientists. The test subjects—people like you and me—ate plain old white bread. The researchers then measured the test subjects' blood sugar responses to get a baseline. They assigned white bread the value of 100. They subsequently fed the test subjects virtually all known carbohydrates at separate times. For each food, they measured the blood sugar of the subjects. The result was the glycemic index. The research has been compiled into glycemic index lists, several of which are available via the Internet and in various books. A value of 20, peanuts, is lowest. Highest is 164 for frozen tofu dessert. Refer to Appendix B for how to obtain the Glycemic Index.

Understanding and Using the Glycemic Index

Foods that have a glycemic index score of 70 or higher are considered high glycemic, foods scoring in the 40 to 69 range are considered moderate glycemic, and foods scoring 39 and below are considered low glycemic. Keep these broad categories in mind; they'll help you avoid memorizing a bunch of precise numbers.

The following is an overview of glycemic indexing that is simple and easy to remember. That way, you don't need to keep a chart in your wallet to eat with confidence.

Here is our ranking of carbohydrates, from worst to best:

1. **Starches.** These include rice, corn, wheat, white potatoes and all foods made from them, bagels, pasta, cookies, cake, muffins, chips, crackers, popcorn, baked potatoes, rice cakes, and such. Remember all those times you ate rice cakes, thinking they didn't have many calories? They don't, but they are ranked as one of the highest foods for stimulating blood sugar (at 110). Oh, dear. Generally speaking, refined starches are considered to be high-glycemic foods.

2. **Sugars.** These include table sugar and most candy. Also included here are honey, molasses, and rice syrup. Sugars are moderate to high glycemic. When reading the label, an ingredient ending in "-ose" indicates a sugar. The glycemic index range is typically 80 to 90.

> **Body of Knowledge**
>
> Although most starches are very high glycemic, barley and imported, long-cooking, steel-cut oatmeal (a hard-to-find item) are unprocessed starches that are low glycemic. Other starches that are moderate glycemic are semolina wheat pasta, basmati rice, and whole-grain breads that don't contain enriched flour and food coloring.

3. **Chocolate.** We just had to give chocolate its own listing. We know you desperately want to know if you should give up your chocolate. Chocolate is moderate glycemic. Dark chocolate is about 63. Milk chocolate and white chocolate are higher because they contain more sugar, but they are still moderate glycemic.

4. **Fruits.** These include most fruits such as apples, grapes, oranges, strawberries, cantaloupe, figs, berries, and pears. Fruits are mostly low glycemic or moderate glycemic. The glycemic index range is typically 40 to 75.

5. **Vegetables.** These include all vegetables except corn and white potatoes, which are high glycemic. Yams and sweet potatoes are considered to be vegetables and not starches. Vegetables are low glycemic. Their glycemic index range is typically 20 to 40.

In summary, refined starches raise blood-sugar levels the fastest and the highest, followed by sugars, chocolate, fruits, and vegetables, the lowest blood-sugar stimulators.

Eating Carbs with Confidence

Yes, you can still enjoy your favorite carbohydrate treats. However, now that you know how these carbs work in your body, you might want to change the way you eat them. As part of your overall food consumption, carbs should be about 35 to 50 percent of your caloric intake. So let's look at each group separately.

We will pass on reviewing chocolate since it is such a limited "food group." The good news is that, yes, you can have chocolate. But don't let it become the primary carbohydrate you eat.

Starches Make Great Condiments

Starches come in two varieties:

◆ Refined starches include white flour, enriched flour, cornstarch, white potatoes, and white rice. The refined starches are nutrient poor.

◆ Complex starches include whole-wheat flour, brown rice, stone-ground wheat, barley, rye flour, and corn on the cob. The complex starches have more vitamins and minerals. You benefit more from eating complex carbohydrates.

> **Thinspiration**
>
> If you are shopping for bread and you want to eat complex carbohydrates, check the label. If it says whole-wheat bread, read the fine print. Make sure the bread doesn't have enriched flour or food coloring in it. Caramel food coloring is often added to make a bread product appear to have more whole grain than it actually contains. Enriched flour is a refined starch. Make sure the first ingredient listed is whole-wheat flour, stone-ground flour, or any whole grain.

Limit your intake of starches. You can tell you have overdone the starches when the waistband of your jeans gets tight in the mid-afternoon or evening. Yes, you get immediate feedback about eating too many starches. The puffy tummy tells you that insulin has been working extra hard. Plus, carbohydrates require water for digestion, so you may also be retaining fluid. There isn't much you can do about the puffy tummy that day, except avoid starches for the rest of the day. But you can learn what not to eat the next day!

The low- to moderate-glycemic grains that you can eat more freely than other starches are barley, semolina pasta, rye, imported long-cooking oatmeal, corn hominy, and wheat kernels.

We suggest you treat the rest of the starches as condiments. What do we mean by a condiment? It's something eaten in small quantities. Let us give you an example: Janet tends to avoid bread, but she loves asiago cheese bread. So she takes part of the loaf and turns it into croutons. She cuts the bread into cubes and sautés them in olive oil and butter with a little garlic. Voilà! Janet has the most delicious croutons for her green salads. A couple of croutons are all it takes to savor that delicious bread taste, and croutons are perfect condiment size.

Another idea is to order sandwiches at the deli the way I once did. I said, "I'll have a ham and cheese, hold the bread." The man behind the counter didn't bat an eyelash. He just looked right at me and said, "I can do that." My sandwich sans bread was terrific. I ate it with a plastic knife and fork, but you could also eat it as a rollup. Roll up the lettuce, tomato, cheese, and ham into a tube and eat. A couple potato chips were my starch condiment. Also, I had a dill pickle. Yum. Don't forget to eat those wrap-type sandwiches with a knife and fork. Cut open the wrap and eat what's inside, leaving behind the wrap.

Some of our clients love pasta so much they center almost every meal around it. A little is fine, a lot makes a person balloon up. Pizza is a family favorite. Our energetic teenage boys love pizza, and they can eat plenty of it just fine. But what's a parent to do? We eat the topping but hold the bread. It's delicious and, with a green salad, truly is a meal made for a thin adult.

By the way, is this wasting food? Think of it this way. The garbage disposal will enjoy it far more than you will when you can't fit into your jeans the next day.

What about all those cookies and cakes and desserts? Again, just eat them as condiments and you will be fine. Eat a small portion that you've left room for, not some giant slice of cake after you've already eaten dinner!

Sugar Is Sweet and Okay to Eat ... Sometimes

Sugars are one notch below starches on the glycemic index because they stimulate blood sugar a bit more slowly than the starches. It's okay to have some sugar. Really. Sugars *aren't* as bad as starches as far as blood-sugar surges; just handle them with care. A spoonful of sugar in tea or coffee is fine, but a bagful of candy is too much. You knew this already because a whole bag would take you way beyond 5 on the hunger scale.

Weighty Warning

Research indicates that eating high-glycemic starches raises your body's triglycerides and increases cholesterol, because you have increased your insulin production. By avoiding high-glycemic foods, you also lower your risk of diabetes. Many diabetics are successfully controlling blood-sugar levels this way.

Body of Knowledge

Most of the time, when people say they are hooked on sugar, they really mean they are hooked on starches that contain sugars. Very few people eat sugar directly from the bowl. Take away the starch part of the cookie and not much is left.

Some people are more dramatically affected by eating sugar than others. If you find that sugar hypes you up, just avoid it as much as you can. If you find that you can't eat just one bonbon and instead end up eating the whole box, you might want to pass up the first one. Most of the time, when you are eating a well-balanced, nutritious diet of proteins, carbs, and fats, your body can handle a bit of sugar. Find out what works for you and your body through experimentation.

Fruit Is Yummy

We are now at the place in the list where you can relax more. Fruits are terrific for you. Enjoy them. As you know, the new dietary guidelines recommend that you eat five or more servings of fresh fruits and vegetables a day. So go for it. Enjoy an orange for breakfast and berries for dinner.

All fruits contain vital *nutrients* and important sugars that your body needs for health. Fruits also are abundant in fiber, which is important for good health and timely elimination.

Make your motto "I haven't met a fruit I didn't like." Of course, eat them 0 to 5— that is, don't overeat them. Fruits are ranked higher on the glycemic index than vegetables, so it is not a great idea to eat five servings of fruit all at once. In fact, it is best to balance those five fruits and vegetables so that you eat about three servings of vegetables and two of fruits.

Veggies for You and Me

You can't go wrong eating vegetables. Think salads (more on salad dressing in the next chapter on fats), broccoli, spinach, and snow peas. Remember cauliflower, celery, and green beans, zucchini, summer squash, and cabbage. And don't forget tomatoes, cucumbers, and radishes. The list goes on and on.

Vegetables are positively packed with health-giving nutrients. They contain lots of fiber plus the phytonutrients that protect us from disease and aid our immune functioning. They contain a wealth of antioxidants to neutralize cell damage that happens in our everyday life. Ounce for ounce, vegetables make a great contribution to your health.

If the glycemic index seems more complicated than you want, consider this. Your stomach is only about the size of your fist when unstretched, give or take

> **Thinspiration**
>
> The next time you want a baked potato, reach for yams and sweet potatoes. They are delicious, plus they are low glycemic. Add some butter and if you like sprinkle with cinnamon or nutmeg. You may find you prefer them to white baked potatoes.

some. In a meal containing protein, carbohydrates, and fats, only 35 to 40 percent of the calories in that fist-size collection of food should be your carbohydrates. Since your carbohydrate intake should include five servings of fresh fruits and vegetables a day, just how much room is left for starches and sugars? That's right, about a condiment size.

Nutrient-Rich Foods

Now we will introduce a concept to help you get the most nutrients from that modest amount of food that fits into the size of your fist. Dietitians call it *nutrient density.* The idea of nutrient density is to get as many nutrients in what you eat as possible. For example, if you want a sweet-tasting liquid, you get more nutrients from the same amount of orange juice as from a soft drink or soda. You get more nutrients from an apple than from a slice of white bread. You get more nutrients from barley pilaf than from white rice, even if it is enriched rice. You certainly get more nutrients from a green salad than from potato chips. You get more nutrients from Romaine or bib lettuce than from Iceberg, which we call "crunchy water."

So, when you are making your selections of carbohydrates, make sure you get as much nutritional power from your food as possible. Do this for your health—and you'll also fit into those jeans.

> **Lean Lingo**
>
> **Nutrient density** describes the extent to which a food supplies all kinds of nutrients—vitamins, minerals, phytonutrients, antioxidants, enzymes, and energy.

But What About My Treats?

Joan is a working mom who tries to eat balanced meals and stay within the 0-to-5 hunger scale. She does fine until it's "time for dessert." She tends to eat her treats regardless of her fullness and regularly ends up overeating. We sympathize. We're talking about treats, after all. We like them and we know you do, too. Because they're quick-acting carbs, treats make us feel good. We know few people who take a fish fillet to bed when their boyfriends don't call. Instead, people prefer treats such as cake, cookies, even mashed potatoes and other comfort foods.

When you want a treat, plan for it in your day's eating. That way, it's included in eating 0 to 5, and it's budgeted into your total carbohydrate intake. Sound challenging or nearly impossible? If you follow eating 0 to 5 closely and eat nutrient-dense foods about 80 to 90 percent of the time, you can have a treat every day. Remember to factor it into the 35 to 50 percent of your total carbohydrate eating.

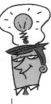

Thinspiration

It's time to rethink treats. Rather than volume, go for quality and eat only the best of whatever you choose. Then make sure you really enjoy it. So, if you want a treat after dinner, and you haven't reached a 5 on the hunger scale, you can have your treat. Just make sure you don't eat above 5. The treat can be what you want—chocolate chips, a bite or two of cheesecake, whatever.

Carbohydrate Loading Is Too Big a Load

Yes, that "too much of a good thing" adage applies to even low-glycemic foods. There's always the temptation to do what is known as "carbohydrate load." Carbohydrate loading is eating too much of even low-glycemic foods. When you do, the high quantity of carbohydrate causes the blood sugar to spike and then the pancreas reacts as if a person ate a smaller amount of a high glycemic food, pumping more insulin into the bloodstream than necessary. The excess insulin causes the body to store fat. So too many low-glycemic carbs can also cause the body to store fat. Some semolina spaghetti is low glycemic, but going back for a second serving could make it high glycemic.

Another way to carbohydrate load is to have too many types of carbohydrates in one meal. For example, semolina spaghetti with tomato and vegetable sauce, a salad with croutons, steamed carrots, and a cookie for dessert would constitute carbohydrate loading. So, too, would a meal of tofu, rice, beans, bread, and pie for dessert. Although each of these items would be acceptable as part of a regular meal, the combination makes for high-glycemic eating.

Even when you eat from 0 to 5, you have to avoid carbohydrate loading if you want to get your best weight-loss results. Remember to balance your meals with proteins and fats. Recommendations for balanced meals are in Chapter 14.

Vegetarian, Not Starch-arian

Some of our clients are vegetarians. At their first weight-loss consultation, when we ask them when they started to gain weight, invariably they answer, "Why, it was when I became a vegetarian."

How can this be? It's because frequently when people become vegetarians, they actually become starch-arians. Rather than eating more vegetables, they radically increase their starch intake. The key to a vegetarian's weight loss is to eat foods that contain high-quality protein and to only eat starches as a condiment. In other words, a vegetarian can't fill up on starches and expect to get to his or her ideal size.

A vegetarian who wants to lose weight can obtain high-quality protein from eating soy-based products (such as tofu, tempeh, soy milk, and soy protein powder) combined with nuts, grains, and seeds. Soy products are classified as a carbohydrate and don't have complete protein. Soybeans have a glycemic index count of 25, which is low. Soy milk is a 43; regular cow's milk is a 39. Tofu frozen dessert is a whopping 164. Power bars are 81 … much higher than dark chocolate.

Because soy products are carbohydrates, they need to be factored into the total carbohydrate consumption and into protein consumption. Vegetarians who eat fish, seafood, poultry, eggs, or cheese have a better chance of getting to their ideal size.

Thinspiration

Here's a tough question: How do you get in the habit of eating fruits and vegetables if you don't normally eat them now? First, eat lots of your favorites. If you love apples, eat them often. If you love a good salad, have one almost every night. Second, try new varieties and prepare your favorites using new recipes. You will quickly learn to make fruits and vegetables a natural part of your diet. Fresh fruits and vegetables are also convenient because most are delicious when raw.

Carbohydrates add delicious variety to our food intake. But they aren't all created equal. Enjoy fresh fruits and vegetables, sugar in moderation, and keep your starch consumption low. Eat starches, if at all, as a condiment, that is, have a taste, not a portion.

The Least You Need to Know

- Carbohydrates include starches, sugars, fruits, and vegetables.

- Glycemic indexing rates carbohydrates by how they raise blood sugar, which can cause the body to store fat.

- For weight loss and for health reasons, eat more low-glycemic carbohydrates and fewer starches.

- Eat starches as a condiment, meaning have a taste or two, not a whole portion because starches are usually high glycemic and cause the body to store fat.

- You can't go wrong eating green vegetables, because they are packed with good nutrition, have plenty of fiber, and are low glycemic, meaning they don't cause the body to store fat.

- If you are a vegetarian, make sure you haven't also become a starch-arian.

Fats Can Make You Thin

In This Chapter

♦ Fats are essential for weight loss

♦ Eat less fat rather than low fat

♦ Your good health depends on eating the right fat

Here's some more good news! Fats are an essential part of getting to your ideal size. They do not, as a friend recently suggested at lunch, go directly from your mouth to the fat cells on your tummy and hips. She intellectually knew this isn't the case, but she had been brainwashed into fearing fats at all costs. What a shame! Of course, anyone who overeats fat could gain weight, but one of the most important things you can do for your weight is to lighten up about fats. Relax and eat the ones that are best for you.

Over and over again, when our weight-loss clients move away from severely limiting their fats and stop eating processed low-fat foods, their stubborn weight starts coming off. So get ready to eat *some* fat and reach your ideal size!

Fats Are Not the Enemy

All experts agree that *dietary fat* is an important component of a healthy diet. What they don't agree on is basically everything else. Some diet gurus advocate eating virtually no fat; others suggest that you eat lots of protein and fat—as long as you avoid carbohydrates. Some tell us that eating saturated fats such as butter gives us high cholesterol, heart disease, and clogged arteries. Others claim that saturated fats themselves are not harmful. Some advocate only unsaturated fats—the liquid oils such as canola oil or olive oil. The food industry now offers us another kind of fat—trans fats.

What's a person to do? Use common sense, learn from the research, and avoid going to extremes. Extremely low-fat diets can produce very unpleasant results. One woman in her mid-30s cut out virtually all dietary fats. She was also an exercise fanatic. Her face became as deeply lined with wrinkles as a 90-year-old woman. Why? Because her body needed at least some fat to keep skin supple.

Your body needs fats for you to release weight and get to your ideal size. By eating the right fats in the right proportions, you can enjoy watching your body fat melt away.

Before we get into some of the nitty-gritty details about dietary fat, let's list some of the known benefits of fat, especially *essential fatty acids* (*EFAs*):

♦ Fat is required for hormones to be manufactured. Without fat, your hormones get out of whack. This includes your thyroid gland and the regulation of women's hormonal cycles, including menopause. Men require optimum hormonal activity for high-energy sex and good muscle mass.

♦ Fats are required for proper insulin function.

♦ Fat is necessary for red blood cell formation.

♦ Fat lubricates your joints.

♦ EFAs regulate the transport of oxygen and energy through your body.

♦ EFAs are essential for the formation of cells, particularly in the nervous system.

♦ EFAs increase your body's metabolic rate.

Lean Lingo

Dietary fats are fats you eat. Body fat refers to the fat your body stores in the adipose tissues of your body. Consuming fat does not necessarily translate into accumulated body fat. Your body can produce body fat from dietary fats, carbohydrates, or proteins. Your body needs **essential fatty acids** (**EFAs**) for important metabolic processes. EFAs are fats that cannot be synthesized by your body; they must be ingested.

Eating fat doesn't make you fat. At least it won't unless you overeat fat-filled foods. So go ahead and enjoy eating some fat without guilt. Don't think of fat as "the forbidden food" because you don't want it to seem too alluring.

Types of Fats

Fats are the most highly concentrated form of fuel. They contain more calories per ounce than either proteins or carbs. Naturally occurring dietary fats are made up of building blocks called fatty acids. Fats come in three basic forms: saturated, polyunsaturated, and monounsaturated. Plus, today there's a fourth type of artificial fat present in food called trans fats. The chemical structure of a fat determines its *degree of saturation*. Most foods contain a mixture of the three basic types of fat, with one type predominating.

Lean Lingo

The **degree of saturation** of a fat refers to its arrangement of carbon and hydrogen atoms. A saturated fat is one that carries the maximum number of hydrogen atoms in its carbon chain. It's "saturated." An unsaturated fat has room for additional hydrogen atoms, which tends to make it more biologically active.

Saturated Fats

Saturated fats come from animal products, including milk and milk products, and from several vegetable sources. Basically, saturated fats are useful only as sources of energy. Their structure makes them easily absorbable into our fat cells. The following are common sources of saturated fats:

Butter	Milk
Cheese	Beef
Lamb	Veal
Pork	Poultry
Lard	Vegetable shortening
Cocoa butter	Palm oil
Coconut oil	Kernel oil
Whipping cream	

Polyunsaturated Fats

Polyunsaturated fats are found in several seeds, seed oils, and vegetable oils, as well as in many types of fish, especially fish that live in cold waters. The following are common sources of polyunsaturated fats:

Corn oil	Safflower oil
Sunflower oil	Soybean oil
Flaxseed oil	Salmon
Mackerel	Herring
Cod	Sardines
Albacore tuna	Black currants
Flaxseeds	Sunflower seeds
Corn	Evening primrose

Monounsaturated Fats

Monounsaturated fats are found in certain vegetable oils and nut oils, which are best when unprocessed. The following are common sources of monounsaturated fats:

Olive oil	Canola oil
Peanut oil	High-oleic safflower oil

Trans Fats

Trans fats are man-made fats created by transforming unsaturated fats into saturated fats through heat and hydrogenation (adding hydrogen atoms). For instance, hydrogenation turns liquid vegetable oils into solids such as margarine and shortening. The food industry likes trans fats because they extend the shelf life of products. However, recent studies show that trans fats may cause serious harm, including increased insulin production, decreased testosterone, lower metabolism, and higher bad cholesterol.

Trans fats are found in commercially available baked goods such as crackers, chips, cookies, pies, and donuts. Notice that trans fats often show up in processed foods that are loaded with high-glycemic carbs that cause insulin to spike and extra fat to be stored. To identify trans fats, check the list of ingredients on a food product and look for the phrases "hydrogenated" or "partially hydrogenated." Then avoid them.

When you eat any of the first three types of fat, consume them in their unrefined and unprocessed states whenever possible. Just as we suggest that you eat unprocessed carbohydrates and proteins, we recommend that you try to eat the fats that are most natural and the least processed. Some of them, such as flaxseed oil, need refrigeration to stay fresh and not get rancid.

> **Body of Knowledge**
>
> Fat helps satisfy hunger in part because it takes longer to digest than carbohydrates or protein. Fat often carries the flavor of food and feels satisfying in the mouth—moist and tender or brown and crispy.

Yes, Fats Are Also Essential

Just as we noted that your body needs essential amino acids and requires certain saccharides for good health, so, too, does your body require essential fatty acids (EFAs.) Your body can't synthesize these from other foods you eat. You must ingest them.

Essential fatty acids are beneficial for hormone production. The brain needs EFAs to function properly, and they are critical for the transmission of nerve impulses. EFAs also aid you in many other ways. They help …

- Improve skin and hair.
- Reduce high blood pressure.
- Lower cholesterol and triglyceride levels.

EFAs are also directly involved in your fat metabolism. Through various biological processes, some EFAs become prostaglandins. One type of prostaglandin, PGE-1, is critical to the proper control of insulin production and indirectly helps burn body fat. Prostaglandins, derived from EFAs, also …

- Act as an antidepressant to control your moods.
- Prevent development of allergies.
- Aid your immune system.
- Reduce inflammation in joints.
- Help move cholesterol through your body.

As you can see, we need our EFAs. In fact, it is a good idea to treasure them. They will help you lose weight. There are two kinds of essential fatty acids: omega-3s and omega-6s.

Omega-3s

Omega-3s consist of docosahexaenoic, eicosapentaenoic, and alpha-linolenic acids. The first two are considered to be the most important omega-3s and are only found in deep-water fish like salmon. Alpha-linolenic acid is found in found in deep-water fish, emu, fish oil, and some vegetable-based oils, including flaxseed and walnut oil.

Omega-3s have become less common in the American diet over the past 50 years ... which is unfortunate. They offer powerful health and weight-loss benefits. They help rev up our fat-burning mechanism.

Omega-6s

Omega-6 fatty acids consist of linoleic and gamma-linolenic acids. They are found in raw nuts, seeds, and legumes and in such unsaturated oils as borage, grape seed, primrose, sesame, and soybean. The omega-6 fatty acids in these oils are destroyed when heated, so they should be consumed in an uncooked and unprocessed form.

How Much Fat Is Too Much Fat?

Studies show that the average American diet consists of about 39 percent fat. Wow! That is more than enough. The American Heart Association suggests we keep our fat intake to 30 percent. Other experts suggest we limit fat to anywhere from 15 to 25 percent.

Consider poor Joan. Her diet was fat-heavy and she never realized it. She thought that by eating low-fat foods she was eating less fat. Most days, Joan had a cup of coffee and a fast-food cheese Danish for breakfast on the way to work. On her good days, she gobbled down a bowl of cereal with milk. For her midmorning snack— obviously she was hungry on such a pitiful breakfast— she ate some low-fat cookies. Her favorite lunch was a cheeseburger and fries, but she also often ate a big salad (loaded with everything they offered at the salad bar). Her family preferred at least one fried food at dinner, and she was more than willing to oblige. Of course, pizza was a regular family fare for busy days. Ice cream was the standard dessert.

Thinspiration

Try to consume a diet containing sufficient EFAs, about 10 to 20 percent of your daily calorie intake. Since these fats can be hard to get from diet alone, we recommend that you consider using supplementation, which is described in the next chapter.

Joan's diet easily drifted into the 40-percent-or-more fat-percentage range. Even when she ate at the salad bar for lunch, she loaded—really loaded—her plate with cheese, mayo-based salads, and dressing (low fat, of course). It wasn't any one thing she ate that was bad. Most items were fine, but her overall diet was fat focused. She never knew it—only her waistline did.

Joan ate too little protein and too many high-glycemic carbs. Even though she often ate low-fat foods, she still ate plenty of high fat foods. Her diet was high in trans fatty acids and low in EFAs. With a little bit of conscious effort, Joan could have adjusted her diet to 30 percent or less in fat. She just didn't realize her problem.

What about you? What will work for your weight loss? What will get you to your ideal size and keep you there?

A good starting point is the American Heart Association guideline. Limit your daily fat intake to 30 percent of all calories you consume. Try to eat even less fat. Limit saturated fats to 10 percent of your total food intake, with the rest of your fat intake coming from monounsaturated and polyunsaturated fats. Consume at least 10 percent, preferably 20 percent, of total calories from EFAs.

This does *not* mean you must count fat grams. In practical terms, just make sure your meals contain protein and lots of the good carbohydrates such as vegetables and fruits. Serve yourself smaller portions of high-fat foods compared to the other foods you eat.

> **Thinspiration**
>
> Eat fats intelligently, not emotionally. You don't need to abstain from food fats, but don't gorge on them either. Fatty foods often appeal to your palate, which is good, but you don't need to eat seconds or thirds at mealtime to feel satisfied.

Eating Low Fat Can Make You Fat

Oh, those low-fat labels! By now you have purchased and eaten processed foods labeled "low fat." The grocery store shelves abound with them. Why? Because you've been told not to eat too much fat. Your choices are amazing: low-fat cheeses, low-fat spreads instead of butter, low-fat mayonnaise, low-fat salad dressings, low-fat cookies, low-fat candy, low-fat ice cream, and on and on. As we said, you can choose these low-fat foods, but please don't. They're making you fat. They are deceiving you and causing your body to store fat.

> **Thinspiration**
>
> Stay away from low-fat processed foods. Search them out in your house and toss them. True, they are low in fat, but they simply can't deliver on the implied promise of a lean trim body.

Any food you eat can only have three nutritional components—protein, carbohydrate, or fat.

When food-processing manufacturers remove fat from foods, usually they replace it with carbohydrates. Often there's more sodium as well, especially in cheese and dairy products. What kinds of carbohydrates are added into the low-fat food? You guessed it. High-glycemic carbs are added. Your body may react to these low-fat foods by spiking blood-sugar levels. The pancreas then goes on alert and overreacts, excreting more insulin than you need to lower blood-sugar levels into the safety zone. Any excess insulin starts storing fat, the very thing you want to avoid.

Less Is More

Here's advice that will shock some of you struggling to lose weight: Please eat real food with real fat, not artificial fat. Buy real salad dressings or, better yet, make your own so that you know it contains only the best unprocessed oils. Purchase butter, real cheese, real mayonnaise, and olive oil and use them when you prepare meals. If you have ever eaten low-fat ice cream, you know how it is. You can eat and eat and never get what you want—that rich, fabulous, decadent taste of the real thing. Yes, you can still keep your fat intake under control when you eat real fat. In fact, you should do better. Real fat gives you a sense of satiety, that feeling that you have eaten well.

If you have a tendency to eat too much fat, however, try this simple approach: Eat less fat. You can have butter but have less butter. Ditto salad dressings, mayonnaise, and so on. Make your portions of red meat smaller. Skip the French fries at lunch. Go for quality, not quantity. If you eat 0 to 5 and concentrate on protein, fruits, and vegetables, you won't need a lot of fatty food to feel satisfied. A little goes a long way. Thoroughly enjoy eating real fat by eating less fat—and watch the body fat come off.

Cholesterol, Fat, and Starch

As you can tell by now, the fat you eat does not directly deposit itself on your hips, belly, and thighs. Dietary fat does many important things to help you release fat stores and maintain high health and energy.

But what about cholesterol? First of all, your body needs *cholesterol*. It is not a fat. If you don't eat enough foods containing cholesterol, your body will synthesize it. Cholesterol is needed for the production of all body hormones. Too much isn't good, but not enough isn't good either.

Dietary cholesterol is not the same thing as blood cholesterol. Recent studies show that the dietary foods that cause high blood-cholesterol readings are the same foods that raise triglyceride levels and can cause the body to store fat. That's right, high-glycemic starches. Should your annual physical reveal a high-cholesterol reading, your doctor will discuss the following factors in your lifestyle and diet:

- Intake of starches

- Intake of other high-glycemic foods

- Alcohol use and frequency

- Amount of dietary fat eaten

- Exercise intensity and frequency

- Body mass index (Are you overweight?)

Lean Lingo

Cholesterol is not a fat but rather a waxy substance. Your body needs a certain amount of cholesterol to synthesize hormones. If you do not consume enough cholesterol, your body will make what it needs.

To lower blood-cholesterol levels:

- Avoid starches and eat low- to moderate-glycemic foods

- Consume alcohol sparingly

- Eat no more than 30 percent fat

- Get plenty of exercise

- Reach your ideal size

Amazing! The first four recommendations are the very activities that will help you reach and stay at your ideal size! Isn't it great that your efforts at weight loss will so powerfully benefit your health and many other aspects of your life?

Weighty Warning

Fast food is the perfect food for gaining weight. It's overly high in saturated fats and trans fatty acids, it's filled with the starches that your body uses to increase fat stores, and it's supersized to give you even more of what you don't need. If you end up eating at a fast-food restaurant, eat only half the bun or throw it away entirely and eat the meat and cheese as a rollup. You will have made the best of the worst. Or you could choose a salad with real salad dressing. Remember to hold the dressing to less than 30 percent of your food intake, so you may want to only eat some of the packet. Drink water.

Fat Shopping and Eating Tips

For some reason, our love-hate relationship with fats inspires confusion and frustration. So here's a list of everyday tips that should help you manage your fat consumption.

The following is a list of what to buy at the store:

- **Olive oil.** The darker the better because it's the least refined or processed and has the most good-for-you oils. If the label says expeller pressed, that's the best kind because it hasn't been heated. Heat turns some of the fats in oils into trans-fatty acids, which have been shown to increase the risk of heart disease.

- **Flax seeds.** They are a great source of omega-3 essential fatty acids (EFAs). You can sprinkle ground seeds on salads, egg dishes, and other dishes.

- **Flax seed oil.** This is useful as a supplement. Make sure it's refrigerated and has lignans added. The benefits of lignans include positive effects in relieving menopausal hot flashes, as well as anticancer, antibacterial, antifungal, and antiviral activity.

- **Salmon.** It's rich in omega-3 EFAs and polyunsaturated fats. Poach or bake more than enough for dinner so that you can enjoy salmon salad—made with real mayonnaise—the next day.

- **Other cold-water fish.** These include mackerel, albacore tuna, sardines, and lake trout.

- **Real versions of anything you have eaten as a low-fat processed food.** We're talking about real ice cream, real salad dressing, real butter, real mayonnaise, and so on.

- **Walnut oil.** An alternative to olive oil for salads.

- **Primrose, borage, and black current oils.** They're high in omega-6 EFAs.

- **Nuts and seeds.** Examples include sunflower and pumpkin seeds. They're also sources of EFAs.

- **An EFA supplement from the health-food store.** This comes in bottles and is refrigerated. It is helpful to supplement essential fatty acids if you aren't eating plenty of salmon, deep-water fish, flaxseeds, walnut oil, and Brazil nuts.

The following is a list of how to cook and eat fats:

- Use olive oil for salad dressings and low-heat cooking. Unfortunately, high heat will destroy olive oil's EFAs.

- Cook with safflower, sunflower, sesame, or corn oils. They're high in omega-3 EFAs and more durable than olive oil.

- Use butter instead of margarine.

◆ Drink whole milk or skim milk if you like milk. Both are fine. Cook with whole milk or cream to get a satisfying taste.

◆ Switch to natural peanut butter that doesn't contain trans fatty acids or added sugar.

◆ Use real cheeses instead of low-fat cheese.

◆ Eat avocados and olives in reasonable portions.

◆ Cook lots of salmon and other cold-water fish. They retain their powerful EFA benefit when cooked.

◆ Choose lean meat cuts or cut all the excess fat off your meat before eating it.

Here are a few tips on how to avoid the wrong fats:

◆ When you purchase processed foods, read the label carefully. If it reads "hydrogenated" or "partially hydrogenated," try to find a substitute. That's another name for trans fatty acids.

◆ Eat modest portions of all fats, especially saturated fats like the kind you find at fast-food restaurants.

> **Thinspiration**
>
> If you want the healthiest salad dressing when eating at a restaurant, ask for olive oil and vinegar. The olive oil is an unsaturated oil and chances are good it hasn't been heated which would create trans-fatty acids, which have been shown to increase the risk of heart disease. If you prefer more flavor, ask for some crumbled blue cheese to go with it.

The Least You Need to Know

◆ Dietary fat is essential for your well-being and attaining your ideal size.

◆ You can eat up to 30 percent of your calories every day as fat, but less may be even better.

◆ Focus on consuming 10 percent of your daily caloric intake as essential fatty acids.

◆ One cause of high cholesterol is eating too many high-glycemic starches, the same foods that cause your body to store fat.

◆ Replace the low-fat processed foods in your kitchen with their real counterparts.

◆ Eating the right dietary fats enables your body to release fat.

Chapter 3

Other Consumables and Supplementation

In This Chapter

- ◆ Other substances you could ingest
- ◆ What artificial foods do for weight loss
- ◆ Supplements to improve your progress

When is a food not a food? Only carbohydrates, proteins, and fats are energy food sources, but you also ingest many other things that don't fall into these three categories.

We want you to know which things definitely to include in your eating, which ones to avoid, and which ones to use with care. You will also learn which supplements can best support your weight loss success.

Nonfood No-No's

You eat plenty of substances that haven't the faintest resemblance to food. Sometimes you eat them because they are hidden in foods, especially processed foods. Sometimes you eat them because you think they will help you lose weight. Some of them are good for weight loss, some are bad, and some are neutral. Additives and artificial ingredients are typically added to foods in very small amounts, but it has been estimated that the average American consumes about five pounds of additives each year. Wow! That's a lot of chemicals. The sections that follow have the rundown on such substances.

Preservatives, Flavorings, and Food Dyes

These substances are man-made, engineered to preserve the grocery shelf life of processed foods, to enhance flavor, or to give coloring. Most of the time, they are the unpronounceable words on the food label. Try to cut out or cut back on processed foods in your diet. We realize this isn't always easy. Because of our busy lives, we have grown accustomed to prepared foods that are ready to be popped into the microwave.

> **Thinspiration**
>
> As best as you can, eat unrefined and unprocessed foods. Your body knows how to digest these. They are the key to life-long weight maintenance. Start reading food labels. Avoid foods that are loaded with artificial ingredients that you can't identify.

However, your overall nutrition will improve, as will your weight loss, if you orient your diet to natural foods—protein, carbs, and fats.

One of our clients, Anita, loves ice cream. As part of her program to manage her eating and her weight, she went to the grocery store to buy natural ice cream. Brand after brand contained unnatural mystery ingredients. She said her hands got quite cold before she found a carton that contained pure food. But it sure tasted good, and it was better for her family.

This brings us to another reason for turning up your nose at these mysterious artificial ingredients. These include such chemicals as sodium nitrite, BHA, sulfur dioxide, sodium sulfite, calcium disodium EDTA, polysorbate 60, calcium propionate, potassium sorbate, ammonium sulfate, sodium propionate, and disodium inosinate. Also included are colors with numbers, such as yellow 5 or 6. The body doesn't know what to make of them.

We all hope or assume that our bodies will simply excrete them and let them pass on through without doing harm, but some experts now think that the body treats such foreign substances as toxins. Unfortunately, the body has another way to deal with toxins in addition to excretion—it stores them in body fat. Recent studies suggest that the body may create even more body fat so that it has more room to store the onslaught of toxins.

A smart strategy is to just say no to artificial anything in your food as best as you can.

Artificial Sweeteners

You should try to pass on artificial sweeteners, too. Try to eliminate aspartame and saccharine from your diet. They are nonnutritive. Ask yourself how many pounds you have lost since you started drinking diet sodas. So, are they working? Most likely not. Here's why.

Recent studies suggest that artificial sweeteners boost insulin by fooling the body into reacting to them like sugar. As you know, this is not good for weight control. The more unused insulin in your bloodstream, the more fat your body stores. If you are hooked on either aspartame or saccharine, it not only can be detrimental to your health, it also can stall and thwart your weight-loss progress. Give up artificial sweeteners.

Find other beverages to substitute for diet sodas and other beverages sweetened with aspartame or saccharin. These artificial sweeteners can cause weight gain and fat storage. Purified water is an excellent substitute.

Another sugar substitute is called Splenda. We don't recommend it either because it contains high-glycemic starches as a filler. Stevia is a very sweet herb from South America that is popular as a sweetener and is available in powder form at health-food stores. It's nonnutritive, but it's neutral in terms of health and weight loss.

> **CAUTION** **Weighty Warning**
>
> The Food and Drug Administration (FDA) has received reports of aspartame being linked to seizures, visual impairment, pancreas inflammation, and high blood pressure, among other disorders. The warning label on saccharine states that consumption is linked to cancer. These artificial sweeteners, as well as monosodium glutamate (MSG), are called "excitotoxins" because they affect the brain in a negative manner.

MSG

Monosodium glutamate (MSG) is considered a flavor enhancer. It actually gives your tongue's taste bud for protein a false positive indication. The glutamine in MSG is what your taste bud senses and tells you that you are eating protein. Of course, the MSG fools you. It isn't protein, but it is added to many foods, especially proteins, to intensify the protein taste and to fool you into sensing that the food has far more protein than it actually has.

Unfortunately, MSG is renowned for causing headaches and other undesirable side effects. Avoid MSG when you can. At Asian restaurants, where MSG usage is common practice, ask for your food to be prepared without MSG. Check food labels for the presence of MSG. It is neutral in terms of actual weight loss, but it certainly doesn't promote health.

> **CAUTION**
>
> **Weighty Warning** _____
>
> Read the labels carefully if you want to avoid mono-sodium glutamate. Look for these other terms for MSG: meat tenderizer, hydrolyzed protein, textured protein, hydrolyzed oat flour, calcium caseinate, sodium caseinate, autolyzed yeast, and yeast extract. MSG is commonly found in fast foods, dairy products, salad dressings, nondairy creamers, sausage and bacon, lunchmeats, canned soups and sauces, cocoa mixes, and veggie burgers.

Alcohol

Alcohol isn't exactly a weight-loss no-no, but we can't fully endorse it, so we include it in this section. Including alcohol in your weight-loss plan requires care and forethought. Since alcohol isn't a protein, fat, or carbohydrate, we don't classify it as a food. In fact, our wonderful internal food processor and detoxifier, the liver, treats alcohol as a poison.

As for weight loss, well, alcohol is tricky. You need to treat it as a food because alcohol changes your hunger numbers. Alcoholic drinks also contain calories. Your body metabolizes alcohol into sugar. What isn't used for energy is converted into fat. Be sure to account for it in your total food intake.

> **Body of Knowledge**
>
> Even one glass of an alcoholic beverage can stimulate your appetite and dull your senses enough that you can't feel your stomach's hunger numbers. Beer, wine, and all alcoholic beverages stimulate the body to increase excretion of the adrenal hormone cortisol. Cortisol is linked to weight gain in the waist and tummy areas.

Alcohol is an appetite stimulant. It can stimulate you to eat more food than you need (that is, to eat above a 5 on the hunger scale). Alcohol is also a depressant, so it can dull your ability to feel your hunger numbers. This means you could overeat because you couldn't feel your stomach hunger sensations.

Alcohol affects each person quite differently. We know one woman who lost seven sizes, from a size 22 to a size 8, and still drank a glass of wine with dinner every night. Find out how it affects you. If you suspect that alcohol is interfering with your weight loss, stop consuming it.

Yes, Have Water

Drinking water is essential for weight loss. Purified water is best. Have a minimum of eight glasses of water a day, more if you are thirsty or when you are exercising. A handy rule of thumb is to have as many ounces of water as your weight in pounds divided by two. If you weigh about 150, you require 75 ounces of water per day, or about nine 8-ounce glasses. There are no acceptable substitutes for water. Herbal teas, coffee, sodas, and other liquids are not the same as water.

Water constitutes roughly 70 percent of your body and is involved in digestion, absorption, circulation, and excretion. It is critical to the transport of waste products out of your body resulting from your digestion and metabolic processes. As you release excess fat, the toxins stored in body fat are released into your body. Water is essential to flush out these toxins and the toxins hanging around in your bladder, liver, kidney, and bloodstream. How much more motivation do you need?

> **Weighty Warning**
>
> You have an increased chance of being chronically dehydrated if you are obese (BMI over 30). This is because the body actually has a lower water percentage the higher your body-fat percentage. You will have more difficulty releasing weight because you are dehydrated. Hydrating your body will help you release fat.

Don't wait until you are thirsty to drink water. When you wait that long, you are already dehydrated. Dehydration can confuse the hunger/thirst mechanism in the brain, making you think you are hungry when in fact you aren't. If you drink water regularly through the day, it will boost your energy, help satisfy your "mouth hunger," and decrease the likelihood that you will experience headaches, muscle aches, food allergies, or acid stomach.

If you find it a challenge to drink enough water, we recommend that you get in the habit of drinking four to eight ounces every hour on the hour. Just do it. The body will absorb smaller amounts like this more easily and will not excrete it as fast—so you'll make fewer trips to the bathroom versus drinking 16 ounces or more at a time!

We recommend that you take a water bottle with you when you are out and about—running errands or attending your kids' soccer games. Sipping on water keeps your energy level higher and allows for clearer thinking.

Can you drink too much water? One dieter e-mailed that she was drinking 30 glasses of water a day. She wanted to know why she hadn't lost any weight. She probably knew the locations of every public restroom within a 100-mile radius of her home, but this huge amount of water wasn't helping her. While we applaud drinking water, it alone can't make you lose weight. Without enough water, however, you will likely inhibit your ability to lose weight. For more about water and hydration, read the section "Electrolytes" later in this chapter.

Drinking Quality Water

By drinking purified water, you reduce your exposure to certain environmental toxins found in tap water, such as chlorine, pesticides, other chemicals, and parasites. Tap water has been shown to contain chemicals from perfumes, prescription medications, caffeine, industrial runoff, and agricultural production.

Tap water purity standards vary from one water district to another. You might want to ask your public water company for its water-quality report to see what you are drinking. For instance, arsenic concentrations vary quite a lot from one part of the country to the next.

Reduce any possible risk to your health by drinking purified water. You can purchase artesian water or purified water at the store, install a water purifier under your kitchen sink, or attach one to the main water supply in your house. Because distilled water is devoid of all nutrients, including valuable trace minerals, we don't recommend drinking it.

Are You a Gum Chewer?

Chewing gum is a habit we hate to call either good or bad. We're not aware of any studies that relate chewing gum to weight loss or gain. It certainly keeps one's mouth and saliva busy, but doesn't seem to aid weight loss or harm it. While we don't think chewing gum is particularly attractive, if chewing works for you, have at it.

Supplements as Support, Not Cure-All

Are pills and powders essential or helpful? You're probably aware of—in fact, you've probably been feeling bombarded by—health claims for certain supplements. TV infomercials, radio stations, newspapers, and magazines are bursting with magical claims for various pills and potions. Kind of confusing and intimidating, isn't it?

The supplements category includes *micronutrients*—vitamins and minerals—as well as protein supplements, oils, and metabolic boosters.

While we doubt anyone has ever lost weight just by taking certain vitamins and minerals, your body needs more nutritional support while you are losing weight. In a sense, losing weight stresses the body. Yes, losing weight is good for your overall health and well-being, but the very activity of releasing fat may cause internal stress of its own.

Lean Lingo

Vitamins and minerals are often referred to as **micronutrients** because your body needs only tiny amounts compared to the four basic nutrients: protein, fats, carbohydrates, and water.

Because your stored fat holds toxins—that's where the body stores them—when you start losing weight, the toxins are released into your body to be processed by your liver and excreted. This takes extra work. When releasing fat, some people report feeling sort of "yucky" for weeks or months as the toxin load in their vital organs increases.

With the right kinds of supplementation, you can decrease the toxin load and feel more energized as the fat flushes out. You may also notice that some of your food cravings diminish or simply go away when you take certain supplements. The supplements we recommend will assist you in both feeling your best and protecting your body. They can increase your stamina and overall energy levels as you get to your ideal size.

Antioxidants

Hooray for antioxidants! The various metabolic processes that break down stored fat molecules release free radicals such as superoxide radicals, hydroxyl radicals, hypochlorite radicals, hydrogen peroxide, various lipid peroxides, and nitric acid. Free radicals can be quite damaging to your health. They've been closely linked to cancer and other serious illnesses.

Enzymes already in your body neutralize the free radicals. Certain phytochemicals in your diet also act as antioxidants that neutralize free radicals or support body functions that do. These include vitamins A, C, and E, beta-carotene, flavonoids, and the mineral selenium. These antioxidants are abundant in the five or more daily servings of fresh fruits and vegetables that you are eating, and some are in the essential fatty acids (EFAs). You also can obtain these antioxidants through supplements.

Thinspiration

Eating fruits and vegetables adds antioxidants that help your body fight the free radicals being released in your body while you're shedding excess fat. The support you get from antioxidants helps you feel better during your weight-loss process.

Vitamins

Vitamins are required for the many metabolic processes that release the energy from the food you digest. Right now, as you are losing weight, you want the most energy possible from your food. B vitamins work together synergistically to boost metabolism, maintain healthy skin and muscle tone, enhance immune functions, and promote healthy cells. Several of the B vitamins are critical to the conversion of fats, carbs, and proteins into energy. If you feel that you could use a boost during this time of physical and emotional changes, consider taking a multivitamin and mineral supplement that supplies a balanced formulation.

B Vitamins for Stress

When you're under stress, your body quickly uses up its B vitamins. Because B vitamins are water soluble, what you don't use in a day or so gets eliminated from your body. This means you need a daily dose of Bs.

How do you get vitamin Bs? All meats—especially organ meats such as liver—contain high concentrations of B vitamins. Next best are fruits and vegetables, especially green leafy vegetables. (You're eating those regularly now, right?) Fish, poultry, eggs, and dairy products also contain some of the different B vitamins. Still, your stressed-out body might not be receiving enough of these stress-fighting vitamins.

Unfortunately, B vitamins are also the hardest to digest and assimilate. They require a fully functioning digestive system every step of the way. If your stomach doesn't secrete enough intrinsic factor, a chemical substance produced by the stomach, you won't be able to absorb B-12. This condition can be remedied by taking liquid or sublingual B-12. These bypass the stomach and are instead, absorbed in the mucous lining of the mouth. If you don't have adequate lactobacillus bacteria in the large intestine, you won't process and assimilate all the B vitamins you need. This can sometimes be remedied by taking a lactobacillus supplement.

B vitamins are included in most multivitamin supplements at your health-food store. If you're concerned that your body won't assimilate B vitamin pills that must go through the digestive system, try liquid B vitamins. You simply put a dropperful or so under your tongue. The vitamins are absorbed sublingually (through the mucous membranes of the mouth under the tongue) and bypass the digestive system.

Get your B vitamins from as many sources as you can—meat, fruits, veggies, fish, poultry, eggs, or supplements—and get them every day.

Weighty Warning

A hundred years ago, it was easier to get the minerals you needed from food. But growing soils have become more depleted in the age of agribusiness. Today, we cannot be sure that our grocery-store produce was grown in mineral-rich soil.

Minerals

You need minerals for maintenance of healthy nerves, tissues, muscle, and bones. You also need them for proper muscle functioning and high metabolism. Chromium, for instance, works with insulin to regulate the body's use of sugars and fatty acid metabolism. Minerals play a role in proper hydration. If your minerals are out of balance, you could be drinking all the glasses of water available in the world and still not be hydrated.

There are two kinds of minerals that your body needs:

1. **Macrominerals** are needed in large amounts. These include calcium, magnesium, sodium, chloride, potassium, and phosphorus. These are in the foods you eat. You also can get them in most multivitamin and mineral supplements. These minerals are essential for you to have the proper electrolyte balance in your body.

2. **Microminerals** are needed in very small amounts in your body. Even though you only need trace amounts—that's why they're often called "trace elements"—they are required for good health. Microminerals include chromium, iron, iodine, cesium, lithium, platinum, selenium, vanadium, zinc, manganese, and boron. Altogether there are more than 70 trace elements that your body needs. You can get them from animal protein and from the five servings of fruits and vegetables. When you are losing weight, be sure to get enough but not too much. See Appendix B for supplement suggestions.

Electrolytes

You must have the proper electrolyte balance in your body to get all the value from the water you drink. Jane, in her 30s, was constantly thirsty and drank water all day long. She carried a water bottle with her wherever she went. When she had her body-fat percentage measured, she was startled to learn that she was dehydrated! How could that be? Jane's electrolytes were out of balance. Basically no amount of water was going to get her fully rehydrated.

You obtain electrolytes from your food, but it's possible to be depleted from sweating due to exercise or heat or from fevers and diarrhea.

Sport drinks contain electrolytes, but many come with a price tag of high-glycemic sugars such as high-fructose corn syrup. You don't want to drink a beverage for electrolytes and in the process trigger insulin to store fat. That wouldn't help much. Select sports drinks made with either juice or fructose, which is a lower glycemic sugar. Our favorites are listed in Appendix B.

Thinspiration

Your electrolytes might need a boost from a sports drink or supplement following strenuous activities such as hiking, biking, exercising, running errands all day ... or something stressful like going to the dentist! These drinks typically have dissolved mineral ions that replenish electrolytes lost from sweating, high activity, or stress.

If It's Green, It's Good

Many people who struggle to lose weight have recurrent yeast overgrowth problems. If you're a woman, you know if you have the obvious vaginal yeast infection. But you can have yeast infections in your bowels, ears, and plenty of other places in your body. Many people struggle with these for years. Some go on the recommended yeast-free diets for years and still have yeast overgrowth. Many take prescription medications continually.

When a person can master the yeast, their weight often is more easily released. Our clients have experienced terrific success by drinking greens formulations. These powders are filled with good-for-you green things such as chlorella, spirulina, barley grass, wheat grass, bee pollen, and other nutrients. In addition to supplying phytonutrients, antioxidants, and vitamins, the drinks make the body slightly alkaline. Since yeast grows best in an acidic body environment, the alkalinity helps kill off the yeast and often lets the pounds come off more easily.

One client baked bread every day and was continually exposed to yeast spores. She had yeast growth throughout her body and on her skin. She didn't want to stop baking bread because it was an activity she did with her husband. So she started taking a greens drink and within a couple of weeks had lost a dress size. Her skin rashes cleared up, as did her yeast overgrowth.

Many experts believe the body is healthiest when slightly alkaline rather than acidic. Mix the greens powder with water, hold your nose if you need to, and drink. Greens drinks we prefer are in Appendix B.

It Went In, But Did It Do Any Good?

The better your digestion, the easier it is to be at your ideal size. Unfortunately, good digestion isn't always a sure thing. Digestion becomes impaired by stress, and our digestive efficiency declines with age. It can also be harmed by other health and lifestyle factors. You don't want to miss one single nutrient from the food you eat. Plus, proper and complete digestion can also reduce cravings. So what can you do?

Body of Knowledge

The better digestive enzymes contain hydrochloric acid betaine (HCl betaine) to aid in digesting proteins. HCl is essential for proper absorption of calcium or iron. Make sure your digestive supplement formulation also includes ingredients that assist with both fat and carbohydrate digestion. The ingredients could include lipase, ox bile, bromelain, papain, pepsin, cellulase, lactase, pancreatin, amylase, and protease.

If you feel that your digestion is not ideal, digestive enzyme supplements can really help. There are many brands and formulations of digestive enzymes, and you want to take one that assists with protein, fat, and carbohydrate digestion. Only take digestive enzymes with meals. Appendix B lists some choices for digestive enzymes.

Balance, Balance, Balance

Yes, supplements can help you make sure you're obtaining all the essential amino acids, necessary sugars, essential fatty acids, and micronutrients. But think of them as "supplements," not as substitutes for good food. They're not a short cut to weight loss. One seminar participant, Alice, admitted she was hoping there were pills she could take so that she could keep binging on the sugars and starches she loved. Too bad that won't work. She deserves praise for her honesty, but she won't be able to release her weight.

Eat a balanced diet as described in Chapter 14 and use the supplements for extra support, not the main course. Recommendations for supplements are in Appendix B.

The Least You Need to Know

- ◆ Avoid eating nonfoods and artificial foods because they do not contribute to overall nutrition and could hinder your weight-loss efforts.

- ◆ Consume alcohol carefully (if at all) because it can stimulate appetite and dull your hunger sensations.

- ◆ Drink at least eight glasses of water a day to assist your body in processing and eliminating fat.

- ◆ Use nutritional supplements to support your body in releasing fat, reduce cravings, and maintain energy levels.

Designing Your Nutritional Weight-Loss Plan

In This Chapter

- ◆ Designing a food plan with plenty of appealing choices
- ◆ The pie chart of your plate
- ◆ Soy shakes: yes, no, or maybe
- ◆ The challenge of vegetarianism

Now that you've gotten this far into the book, you're probably thinking, "So, when do we eat?" You've learned a lot of detailed information about how your body works, nutrition, and factors affecting weight. Now you want to put it all together into a weight-loss eating plan that works for you.

Your eating approach must be practical. An unrealistic, idealized system might help you for a few weeks, but you won't likely maintain it. Your weight-loss approach needs to fit the way you really live, taking into account your work, children, family, exercise, recreation, and food preferences. Anything less won't get you to your ideal size for life.

You Need to Like What You Eat

First and foremost, choose foods you like. If you don't like the food you eat, you won't be able to enjoy it and eat beautifully and sensuously. In the preceding four chapters on nutrition, you learned about the nutritional value of a great many different foods. Plus, it's pretty straightforward to identify the benefits of specific foods we didn't list. For instance, we indicated some of the cold-water fish species that are good for you, but you can generally infer that other cold-water fish will have many of the same benefits.

Thinspiration

Only eat food that you enjoy. You do not need to eat unappealing foods to get to your ideal size, nor should you. Make your eating a pleasurable and sensuous delight.

So eat the specific foods that really appeal to you. No, we're not encouraging you to make a quart of ice cream your dinner. But we do mean this: If you have never met a green pea that you like, don't eat green peas. Ditto for cauliflower or onions. Eat foods you do like that have comparable nutritional value.

How many oddball diets have you read about or maybe experimented with? Shellie, age 48, was a classic obsessive dieter. Over the years, she tried special diets that promoted the following:

- Rice cakes (She called them "cardboard sandwiches.")
- Grapefruit ("An orange with a sour disposition.")
- Yogurt ("Milk that's gone bad.")
- Watermelon ("Lots of water, lots of sugar, where's the food?")
- Cabbage soup ("Not bad for the first 20 bowls.")

It took considerable effort to persuade Shellie that she could lose weight and actually eat what she liked … including chocolate. Shellie, now 20 pounds lighter, makes her dieting past sound funny, but her story is all too common. As you know by now, in your efforts to get to your ideal size, no plan will work for a lifetime if you have to eat yucky foods. Shellie still likes watermelon, just not bowls and bowls of it. Too much of even a good thing is not a good thing.

Balance Is Everything

A friend born and raised in France but now living in the United States made this observation: "What amazes me about Americans is that they eat the same foods day after day. Why, in France, we wouldn't think of eating the same food twice in the same week." (As you probably know, the French don't have anywhere near the overweight and obesity issues plaguing the U.S. population.) We like her philosophy of eating a wide variety of foods. This reduces boredom of the palate and also gives a person many more types of nutrients from their foods.

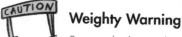

Weighty Warning

Research shows that eating the same types of food day after day can bring on food allergies—one more good reason to eat a wide variety of foods.

The Balanced Meal Pie Chart

For your long-term weight-loss success, it's the ratio of fats to carbs to proteins that's the key. Every meal and, ideally, every snack you eat should contain the following proportions of calories consumed:

- Fats: 30 percent or less

- Proteins: About 25 to 35 percent

- Carbohydrates: About 30 to 50 percent (of these, about half need to be from vegetables and fruits)

- Artificial foods: Avoid if possible

Your Plate

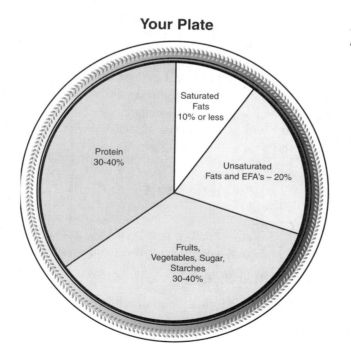

How your plate should look: a balanced meal.

Here's a simple visualization to guide you in eating protein. A healthy portion of most proteins—including fish, beef, pork, eggs, cheese, and poultry—will be about the size of a deck of playing cards. It will contain about 15 to 20 grams of protein.

The Balanced Plate

You could figure out the proportions by counting calories, but we don't recommend doing this. It's boring and can make eating dull and lifeless. We prefer the simpler approach of looking at the composition of foods on your plate. If you balance the proportions of food on your plate by type, you will closely match your nutritional needs. Your protein and fat foods will take up about 50 to 60 percent of your plate; the rest will consist of carbohydrates. Of course, you've got to figure in any side salads, breads, and desserts, but we've found that the plate-balancing approach will keep you from loading your plate with high-glycemic starches.

Improving Your Real-World Food Choices

We like flexibility, but we also know that your weight-loss food plan won't work if you become *too* flexible. You will need some discipline to make it work. Certainly, it's okay to eat less than 30 percent fat and more protein, but make sure you get at least 30 percent carbohydrates, mostly from vegetables and fruits instead of starches. Most starches are high-glycemic and cause the body to store fat. Eat starches in very small amounts to avoid this happening to you.

Thinspiration

Remember that eating the right balance of foods never, never gives you the green light to overeat. You still need to eat according to your internal hunger urges, eating only from 0 to 5. Start eating when you're hungry; stop eating when you're satisfied but not full or overstuffed. Eating too much of good-for-you foods is still overeating.

So let's get real. Let's use these ratios to examine some really bad choices and some really great choices. You will begin to see how you can enjoy wonderful foods and still stay within the guidelines that will help you lose weight.

Lunchtime Meals

Let's take a look at how similar lunchtime meals can go from bad to best by substituting certain foods for better-balanced nutrition and weight loss.

Bad choice:

Double cheeseburger with white bread bun
French fries
Milkshake or soft drink

This meal has enough protein in the cheese and meat, but the rest is pure high-glycemic carbs and trans fats. The obvious question is where's the veggies?

Good choice:

> Double cheeseburger, hold the bun
> Small salad with a bit of dressing
> Apple

You get plenty of protein, and the meat and cheese supply the fat. The salad adds good carbs, as does the apple. The bit of salad dressing adds some taste and some fat. This menu is okay and includes two servings of your daily five fruits and vegetables.

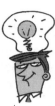

Thinspiration

You have the power to choose what you eat. Use it! You don't need to clean your plate, so pick and choose, making sure you eat the basics: high-quality protein, fruits and veggies, and fats.

Dinner on the Run

In busy families, the temptation to eat high-glycemic starchy foods is great. You may not have the time or energy to fix carefully planned healthy meals. All is not hopeless! A little creativity can go a long way.

Bad choice:

> Pizza and coke

A *huge* number of families eat pizza regularly, as often as once a week. Yours may be one of them. We want you to fit in with your family and not create tension about your eating versus theirs. There are creative ways to eat better—and maybe inspire your family to eat better—even when you're having pizza or some quick alternative.

Good choice:

> Pizza topping, hold the bread and crust
> (eat the topping, leave the crust)
> Salad with dressing of olive oil and
> vinegar or lemon juice
> Carrot or celery sticks

Fortunately, pizza-delivery restaurants often offer salads, or you can make a quick one at home. Add your own healthy, homemade dressing and make carrots or celery available for

Thinspiration

If you give up soft drinks, which we encourage you to do, quit buying them for the kids. Let them decide if they want to spend their allowance money on junk foods and drinks. This may cut down on the amount they consume.

everyone as a side munchie. (You'll be surprised at how often they get eaten.) If you've just gotta have that pizza crust, limit yourself to one slice. This is a good compromise meal. You enjoy eating with the family, you're consuming an adequate amount of high-quality protein, and a salad gives you one or two servings of veggies, depending on the size of the salad.

Don't try to force the whole family to follow your food regimen on pizza night, especially if teenagers are involved. Such well-intentioned preaching is wasted breath. It's better to provide good choices with the pizza and limit the number of times pizza is ordered.

Family Dinners to Live By

For family dinner, plan to offer the two Vs—variety and vegetables. Family dinners need to include a variety of choices so you get a good balance. Sometimes dinners become focused around one item only, and if that item is something starchy like pasta, you're more likely to overeat and consume a nutritionally poor meal. Plan some variety into every meal. One key is to include vegetables that you like. Here are a few other dinner tips:

- Make sure you're including a high-quality, complete protein.
- Include two vegetables.
- If you don't want to cook a second vegetable, have a cold side vegetable such as celery, carrot sticks, or tomato slices.
- Serve only one low- to moderate-glycemic starch at a meal, if at all.
- Skip the bread if there's already a starch included.
- Don't drink your calories at dinner; eat them.
- Avoid artificially sweetened drinks that stimulate appetite.

Thinspiration

Serve dinner from the stove, not family-style with bowls of food at the table. This will discourage overeating and will encourage more controlled eating based on feelings of real hunger and fullness. This may clash with family tradition, but try it and see if it doesn't help limit unconsciously eating second and third helpings.

Here are two possible dinner choices, both very different in how they will affect your weight loss progress. The high starch meal is a poor choice and is drastically out of balance. The second choice is well balanced and delicious.

Bad choice:

> Fettucini alfredo
> French bread

This is a white meal, filled with highly refined wheat products and no high-quality protein. Without proteins and vegetables, you're eating a very high-starch, high-glycemic meal that has a good chance of ending up as stored fat in your body.

Excellent choice:

> Small steak
> Green salad with vinegar and olive oil dressing
> Broccoli
> One small scoop of real ice cream

Even with the scoop of ice cream, this meal is superior. The olive oil provides you with good monounsaturated oil, and you're consuming about 15 to 20 grams of high-quality protein. You're eating two servings of vegetables and, for dessert, natural ice cream. Your proportions stay in balance and the food is yummy. Just eat small portions and stop when you reach 4 or 5 on the hunger scale.

Note: At no time do we encourage you to eat a dressing or food labeled "low fat." You don't need to. If you're concerned about your overall fat intake, avoid foods labeled low fat and eat smaller portions of real fats instead.

Another excellent choice:

> Shrimp Creole (containing tomato sauce, onions, green peppers, celery, and more)
> Hold the white rice (or substitute brown or basmati rice)
> Tomato, cucumber, and onion salad with homemade dressing
> Sautéed cauliflower and zucchini
> A piece of dark chocolate

Here you get superb flavors. You are eating low glycemic, and you get enough protein, veggies, and acceptable fats.

You could also use walnut oil or flaxseed oil on your salad to get EFAs in this meal. The chocolate is a treat that fits in fine.

A note on chocolate here: New, hot-off-the-press (although it won't be hot off the press by our publication date!) research indicates that cocoa powder and dark chocolate increased test subjects' levels of HDL, or good cholesterol. Chocolate contains fatty acids that don't raise cholesterol levels. Also, chocolate doesn't cause acne, isn't addictive, doesn't cause tooth decay, and doesn't interfere with calcium absorption.

Breakfasts of Champions

Poor breakfasts are the downfall of many of us, so don't beat yourself up if you've tended to eat poorly in the morning. You *can* do better, and you will definitely be happier and thinner when you do. For most of us, the key is to include protein and fruits into our hurried morning lives.

Bad choice:

> Cold packaged breakfast cereal and milk
> (or yogurt and granola)
> Orange juice

Another bad choice:

> Danish or muffin
> Coffee

Both of these meals are lacking in enough high-quality protein to keep your metabolism high all day. Plus they are high in the fattening high-glycemic carbohydrates. The orange juice is good, but eating a real orange would be even better. An orange has more fiber and also more nutrients such as bioflavinoids.

Excellent choice:

> Scrambled eggs
> Slice of leftover meat from last night's meal
> Orange
> Water

Some experts consider eggs to be the perfect protein. This breakfast features plenty of protein with the eggs and meat. The orange gives you great value from your carbs. There is some fat in the eggs and meat and also the butter you cooked the eggs in.

Another excellent choice:

> Salmon salad made with real mayonnaise
> Leftover green salad or green beans
> Berries

We're including this "leftovers breakfast" to suggest that dinner foods from previous meals offer a no-cooking way to eat a nutritious breakfast. This breakfast has essential fatty acids—omega-3s—in the salmon, and the real mayo avoids the trans fatty acids. The salad and the berries give you plenty of fiber and are great carbohydrates to eat for breakfast.

Snacks Should Be Nutritious, Too

Betsy and her husband, Dick, are in their mid-40s. Not long ago, they were vacationing in a city new to them and sightseeing a lot. The first afternoon, for a quick snack, they gobbled down delicious cookies from a sidewalk vendor. Within an hour, they were both tired and hungry again. The next afternoon, they actually ate a sitdown snack at their hotel restaurant. For a special treat, they ordered liver pate with dill gherkins and French bread. The snack was delicious. Even better, they had the energy to dance all night (well, at least until midnight!).

The moral of the story: Make your snacks as nutritious as your meals. At a minimum, make them as nutritious as you can.

Here are some snack ideas:

- Peanut butter (ditto almond and cashew butters). Eat it with a spoon or with celery, sliced apples, peaches, or other fruits or veggies.

- Nuts and seeds, whatever kinds you like.

- Pâté, meats, fish, hard-boiled eggs, and cheeses with fruit or veggies. As you can see, we think it's a good idea to cook too much meat at meals so that you have some leftovers for snacks. Also, keep cans of albacore tuna and salmon in your cupboard. That way you have high-quality protein when you need it.

- Celery, carrot sticks, olives, avocado.

- Healthy chips or whole-grain crackers with protein (tuna, peanut butter, and so on).

Thinspiration

We travel with spare protein. Really. We board airplanes with those little cans of tuna or sardines, as well as dried fruits or nuts, just in case we are served unacceptable food or, worse, none at all! A healthy snack keeps the ravenous hunger away that can later lead to overeating. Plus, we hate to be without food!

Simple Approaches Yield Maximum Satisfaction

As you can see, you can eat really well and get full flavor and pleasure from your eating. We avoid the high-glycemic carbohydrates and strongly favor fruits and veggies over starches. Hopefully, you can use these examples as a guide to prepare wonderful meals that include your favorite proteins, vegetables, and fruits in ways that balance your nutritional needs.

Don't worry if changing your habits takes time. It took us a while to get the hang of good eating habits. Over time, however, it was easy to give up the bowl full of rice with a scattering of vegetables. Cutting back on large quantities of breads and pastas was hard but worth it in waist inches lost. Just as important, we found that the high-quality protein boosted our energy so much we never want to go back. The weight stays off, too.

The Trials of a Strict Vegetarian Diet

Vegetarians often struggle with weight. If you have chosen to be a vegetarian but eat cheese, dairy, eggs, and fish, you can use the preceding meal ideas by substituting one of these for the meat suggestions. Cheese, eggs, and fish are high-quality proteins that can be prepared in innumerable ways. Just make sure you emphasize vegetables and fruits. If you are a total vegetarian or vegan, however, meaning you eat no animal products, your protein choices are far more limited. Getting enough high-quality protein is challenging, if not impossible.

CAUTION

Weighty Warning _____

Recent studies suggest that women who eat low-quality protein, such as beans and rice, do not lose weight because the thyroid reacts as if the body is starving. Recent studies also report some concern about possible health risks associated with eating high amounts of processed soy, such as thyroid and hormonal imbalances. So be careful with your soy powders and with protein bars that are high in soy protein isolate.

Many vegetarians consume soy products as their primary source of protein. Unfortunately, soy is not a complete protein because it doesn't have all the essential amino acids, specifically methionine. To get complete protein, soy products need to be eaten with grains through food combining. Even with food combining, consuming 25 to 30 percent protein and only 30 to 40 percent carbs will be a challenge.

Since soy products contain very little fat, be sure to add essential fatty acids and other expeller-pressed oils, such as olive oil and walnut oil, to your intake. Eat plenty of the low- to moderately glycemic fruits and vegetables—and watch those starches!

Soy Shakes as Meal Replacements

Soy shakes are popular as convenient meal replacements for losing weight. They are convenient, but will they give you the results you want? We want to give you the pros and cons of soy shakes and let you make up your own mind. Soybeans in their natural state are green and look like a cross between a snow pea pod and a green pea pod.

Soy powder is a highly refined food product that bears no resemblance to the bean itself.

Before you consider using soy protein powder as a food, determine whether …

1. You have an allergic reaction to soy. (This is a common allergen.) If so, avoid soy.

2. You digest it well. If soy gives you gas, belching, or bloating, we suggest you avoid this food, as you would any food that gives you an unpleasant reaction.

For a soy shake to be a good meal replacement, it should contain …

1. Enough protein for a meal. Therefore, the shake needs to have 15 to 20 grams of protein. Because soy protein is not a complete protein—that is, it does not have the full range of essential amino acids—you need to have a food containing a complementary protein, either at the same meal or during the same day.

2. Low-glycemic carbohydrates and sweeteners only. You don't want a shake loaded with high-glycemic carbohydrates that causes your body to store fat. Avoid soy products with high-fructose corn syrup, maltodextrin, Splenda, or sucrose. Look for fructose or stevia.

3. No artificial ingredients such as artificial sweeteners, food coloring, and preservatives with long chemical names.

4. Enough nutrition to satisfy you without getting hungry again soon. It should keep you from reaching 0 on the hunger scale for about three hours. If you get hungry soon after drinking the shake, it wasn't a meal replacement. You may need to add some high-quality animal protein, some milk, or some fat to your meal so that it gives you enough energy to last you for three hours.

Soy shakes do not offer fresh fruits and vegetables, so you will need to add them to the meal or to other meals and snacks. Soy shakes don't contain much fat, if any, so you need to add fat to the shake. Consider adding flaxseed oil or other omega-3 or omega-6 essential fatty acids.

Some shakes offer the following:

1. Flavorings such as chocolate, vanilla, and strawberry. Make sure they do not use artificial flavorings and food colorings.

2. Added vitamins and minerals.

Select your commercial brand of soy shake based on these criteria. Even better, make your own.

Body of Knowledge

Protein bars are in the same category as soy shakes, but with a couple of differences. They are usually high glycemic, so they should never be considered to be a meal replacement but rather eaten as a candy bar. Next, they may be artificially sweetened. Avoid these bars and select the ones with natural sweeteners. Eat protein bars as you would a candy bar, that is, as an occasional treat after a meal, definitely not as a meal.

How to Make Your Own Soy Shake

Put $1/3$ cup of plain soy powder into a blender. Add a liquid—water, milk, or yogurt. If you prefer, add some fruit and maybe some flaxseed oil. Blend and drink.

For variety, add nut butters, vanilla, or cocoa.

For high-quality protein, consider also eating a hard-boiled egg or some meat or fish for your meal.

Many people also substitute whey powder for soy powder in their shakes. One good reason is that whey powder contains complete protein.

Weighty Warning

Be sure not to overeat soy shakes. Drink only enough to get you to 5 on the hunger scale and no higher. There is a strong temptation to finish a shake even if you are already at 5. A leftover shake is certainly not much of a taste treat. Remember, overeating any food will cause you to gain weight.

Become Soy Wise, Not Fanatical

We question whether it is advisable to drink a soy shake every day because it does not give you high-quality, complete protein. Also, eating the same food every day does not vary your diet. A soy shake once every couple of days is plenty. Remember, they are not going to make you lose weight, just as no other single food can make you lose weight.

The recent research about how soy disrupts hormones deserves careful scrutiny. Stay up-to-date on these studies and, if there comes a time when the evidence is highly conclusive against soy, find another way to get quick meals.

Will Protein Bars Power Your Weight Loss?

Protein bars are often touted as good for weight loss. The advertisements claim that they provide ample protein, nutrition, and oodles of energy all in one convenient package. But will they help you lose weight? The bars are basically a combination of starches, sugars, and protein powder. Read the label to determine the following:

◆ Does it have protein and how much? The best will have more than 10 grams of protein, most likely from soy or whey powders.

◆ Does it have artificial sweeteners such as aspartame and saccharine? If so, take a pass. Do not eat them.

Because even the best protein bars include a blend of starches and sugars, most likely they are high glycemic. We suggest that you consider them to be of limited value for losing weight, about as valuable to your weight loss as a candy bar. You can eat one occasionally as a snack, but any apparent energy boost you get might be from the high-glycemic starches that can cause weight gain. If you do occasionally eat them, make sure you do so using the 0-to-5 hunger scale. Try to find other, healthier snacks.

The Least You Need to Know

◆ Eat balanced meals consisting of foods that you enjoy.

◆ Eat no more than about 30 percent fats, 40 percent protein, and 30 percent carbohydrates at every meal and snack.

◆ Create meals that let you enjoy the health benefits of your food. Eat high-quality protein, essential fatty acids, and low- to moderate-glycemic carbohydrates such as vegetables and fruits.

◆ If you are a vegetarian, follow the nutritional guidelines for eating a balanced diet, making sure you get enough high-quality protein and avoid being a "starch-arian."

◆ Choose soy shakes carefully and drink them occasionally, not as daily meal replacements.

Part

Exercise Is Your Friend

Exercise is one of the most inexpensive yet luxurious of life's pleasures. It helps you lose weight and is a significant factor in keeping your weight off. It lifts your moods and makes you feel good all over.

So what's not to like about exercise? How about that it takes time and energy and feels like work, plus you are "supposed" to do it.

This part of the book shows you how to do exercises that count the most toward getting in shape, and how to enjoy every sweaty moment.

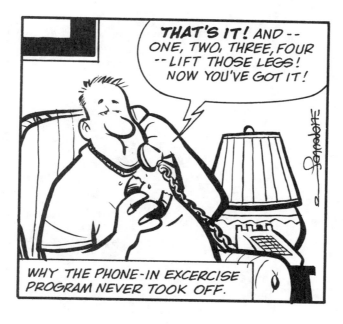

Your Body Wants to Move

In This Chapter

- Overcoming sedentary inertia
- Maintaining your ideal size
- Why you should work at working out

Do you know what modern man is really good at? Sitting. We've really mastered the art of sitting. After all, it's a lot more comfortable to watch television sitting down, and watching television is our national pastime! And that's only part of our regular sitting routine. There's also driving to work, working at a desk, and sitting down for meals. In fact, most golfers even sit in little carts from one hole to the next.

What was once a necessary part of our ancestors' survival—movement—is pretty much optional today. Of course, there's a price to pay for becoming a sedentary nation. We're also getting flabbier. Our muscles maintain their shape from use. The less we use them—and it doesn't take a lot of muscle power to sit—the less shapely our muscles become. It's that simple.

But you already know this, right? So why don't you use your muscles more? For a thousand reasons, we're sure. Everyone can come up with oodles of reasons *not* to exercise. In this chapter, we ask you to take a fresh look at exercise, put aside your well-entrenched prejudices, and commit to a plan to exercise regularly and happily for the rest of your life.

Overcoming Exercise Inertia

Amidst the busy life you live, sometimes exercising is the last thing you want to do. You're tired. Your to-do list is packed with a dozen other things to take care of. Just the thought of exercising makes you exhausted! We know the feeling, too. Some days we have to force ourselves to exercise, but we do it. We do it because we know what happens when we don't, but mostly we enjoy it!

Inertia Has a Price Tag

Overcoming exercise *inertia* is a critical step toward reaching your ideal body size. When we don't exercise, all kinds of unpleasant side effects occur. Our legs get flabby, our waists become bigger, and our upper arms jiggle like Jell-O. We struggle to find enough energy to get through the day. We seem to become more anxious and perhaps a bit depressed. Often these feelings lead us right to the kitchen and directly to the refrigerator.

When we don't exercise regularly, we feel like, well, like slugs. And that doesn't feel good. We like ourselves less. Even our postures sag.

This is probably not the image you want for yourself. Right? Your ideal self-image is instead loaded with positive attributes—great posture, bright eyes, firm upper arms, and a flat tummy. Well, the road that takes you toward your ideal body size involves exercise along the way. In other words, plan to exercise regularly to get what you want.

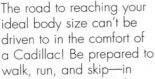

> **Lean Lingo**
>
> In physics, the law of **inertia** states that a body in motion tends to stay in motion and a body at rest tends to stay at rest. The same is true for a person and movement. Thus, according to this law, a person who exercises tends to do more activity overall, and a person who is sedentary tends to stay among the couch potatoes.

> **Thinspiration**
>
> The road to reaching your ideal body size can't be driven to in the comfort of a Cadillac! Be prepared to walk, run, and skip—in other words, to exercise—along the way.

Positive Self-Talk About Exercise

Many people tell themselves that they hate to exercise. This kind of negative internal self-talk is sure to make matters worse. As we've suggested throughout this book, your mind is your most powerful tool to help you reach your ideal size, so use it wisely when it comes to exercise. Don't talk about or even think about exercise in negative terms. Instead, tell yourself the following:

"I love to exercise."

"It feels good to exercise."

"I would rather exercise than sit around at night."

"I love to take walks during lunch."

"I love to go out dancing."

"I enjoy going to the gym and working out."

"I enjoy my aerobics classes."

"I like to play tennis, golf, racquetball, and so on."

"I enjoy my home exercise program."

"I smile after a good workout."

The more you can program yourself to enjoy exercise, the less you have to force yourself to get out and move.

Dealing with Your Barriers

Of course, it's not just negative thoughts that keep you from exercising. You have *real* reasons not to exercise, right? Let's think about them and see if you can get past them.

No Time!

I don't have time to exercise. Of course you don't. We've found that basically no one has time to exercise. We've never had anyone tell us they became regular exercisers because they were bored and didn't have anything else to do. Exercise just seems so frivolous when there are so many other "important" things that must get done.

Maybe your view needs to broaden. Without enough regular exercise, you're much more likely to lack the energy and stamina to tackle all your chores, to feel good at the end of the day instead of exhausted, and to reach your ideal size.

There is no way around your need to exercise. You can't hire someone to do it for you. You can't have it done to you passively while you rest. You can't do just a little and expect huge results. You can't speed it up and do it in less time. Exercise takes as much time as it takes.

Thinspiration

Try this. Exercise 20 minutes for every hour you watch television, play video games, or enjoy other sedentary pastimes. That's just a 1-to-3 ratio. You can even exercise *while* you're watching TV! We're betting you'll learn to enjoy exercising at least as much as viewing the typical TV show. You know that if you have time to watch TV, you have time to exercise at least some.

If you're really struggling to find time to exercise, get creative. When Helen was a mom with a six-month-old, she would head to the park with her baby in the stroller. There she would run circles on a wide path around the stroller so she could get in her running. Undoubtedly she may have gotten a few curious stares from onlookers, but it worked.

Today, most health clubs offer childcare, so you can still get in a workout. Or you could develop a home program if you've got small children. Exercise during naptime, when they're in the playpen, or while they play at your feet. You'll find it worthwhile even if it's not your ideal. And don't forget your spouse! Ask him or her to baby-sit while you work up a sweat and enjoy exercising for a half hour.

> **Thinspiration**
>
> There really aren't shortcuts to exercise. Perhaps that's the real beauty of it. Could it be that your exercise time is time just for you? Time to de-stress, to decompress, to be alone with your thoughts? Time to enjoy some of the sensuous pleasures of your body's movement and sweat?

Put it on your schedule. Don't rely on "when you feel like it" exercising. Schedule exercise into your daily agenda and make sure you block off at least 45 minutes three times a week—or more. Plan to schedule exercise for the rest of your life. Intermittent bursts of exercise are okay, but they don't add up to much over your lifetime. You never outgrow your need for exercise.

What About My Hair!

I hate what exercising does to my hair! Unless you're bald or you shave your head, there's a good chance that working up a sweat will mess up your hair. Yuck! Wouldn't it be great if you could exercise hard without wrecking your hairstyle or needing to shower afterward?

This problem can only be tackled through practical measures and a good attitude. The best attitude to adopt is that *not* exercising wrecks a heck of a lot more than exercising ever can. Not exercising can wreck your weight-loss progress, lower your metabolic rate, and erode your health. So what's a hairstyle and more antiperspirant when we're talking about your ideal size and health?

Carefully choose the type of exercise and the timing of your exercise to handle your showering and hair concerns. Many of us prefer to exercise in the morning before work. Some prefer after work. Noontime aerobics classes are a bit harder for handling personal hygiene, but you can solve the problem if you're motivated enough. How about an easier-to-manage hairstyle?

Embarrassed at the Health Club

Do health clubs intimidate you? Do you find yourself comparing other bodies to yours? Do you believe that others at the gym are looking at your body critically, especially if you're not yet at your ideal size? Or even if you are? We have clients who are embarrassed to be seen riding their bicycles in public. They feel that every passerby is commenting on the size of their thighs. This is real and can be a challenging situation. So how do you overcome this?

We certainly don't recommend hiding out because you aren't in the shape or at the size you want to be. You can start your exercise program at home. There are terrific exercise videos, and home exercise equipment can be a great investment … if you use them (check out Appendix B for more information). Chapter 18 will show you how to set up an at-home exercise plan. You can also join a health club or go to the rec center and exercise. Just be sure to not compare your body to others; rather, use the time as your personal time for you. Luxuriate in the pleasure of moving your body, the sweat, and the heavy breathing.

By all means, do as much exercise out of doors as you want. If a passerby has thoughts about your body, well, only you know how mistaken and petty that person is. He or she is passively riding in a car; you, on the other hand, are getting fresh air, sunshine, and terrific body movement.

Exercise Is Hard and It Hurts

Yes, we don't disagree. At first, you can be stiff and sore after an especially energetic workout. It can be hard to catch your breath, your lungs can feel as if they can't get enough oxygen, you can feel really out of shape. In this situation, you only have two choices—stay out of shape or get in shape.

The only way out is to go through it. You can go slower and let your body build stamina and muscle strength without so much huffing and puffing, wheezing, and stiffness.

Last year, Lucy moved to a small city within 15 minutes of the mountains and great hiking trails. "I thought I was in great shape until I started hiking. Oh my gosh, after a half hour my legs were mush, and they wobbled. My heart pounded. I got woozy but didn't want anyone, namely my husband, to know. After several hikes, he started watching me more carefully. When my legs started trembling as I climbed, he made me stop and take my pulse rate. [Do this by counting the pulse on your wrist or neck for 6 seconds and multiply by 10.] If my heart rate was too high, say over 140, he had us turn around and head down the mountain. I didn't like this because I wanted to get higher up. However, by not pushing myself to the top early on, over the summer, I developed the stamina to go farther and farther every hike. Now those same hikes feel like a cakewalk."

Muscle soreness and stiffness on the days after exercise is caused by a build up of lactic acid in your muscles. To feel better, we recommend drinking lots of water, stretching, and/or Epsom salt baths. You can tell by now that we recommend baths for almost any condition. The luxury of massages is great, too.

The Value of You

Regular exercise isn't just about the many benefits; it is about the value of you. Just what is your value to yourself, your family, and the world? As you value yourself and your contributions, you understand that taking care of yourself is essential to giving to others. Just a note here: If you are a caretaker or are in a care-giving career, it is very important that you take care of you. Many overweight people are primary caregivers and forget to also care for themselves.

Demonstrate your own self-esteem and self-worth by taking good care of yourself through exercise.

Boost Your Metabolism

Exercise boosts your metabolic rate. As you exercise, you increase your muscle mass. Simply by doing this, you have a higher metabolic rate. This means you burn through your food faster. Thus, you actually need to eat more food to stay at your ideal size.

For example, let's compare two women. Both are the same age and weigh the same. The first woman works out by doing strength training three times a week. The other doesn't do any form of strength training. The first woman needs to eat more calories to stay at her ideal size than the other one—simply because she has more muscle and less fat on her body.

This is why. A pound of fat requires only three calories per pound for maintenance. A pound of muscle requires 35 to 50 calories per pound. It is highly beneficial to your weight loss to have a low body fat percentage and high muscle mass.

As we counsel our weight-loss clients, it is amazing how some of them need such little amounts of food while others need more. The amount of body fat as compared to muscle makes a big difference in how much food it takes to stay at your ideal size. It is difficult to realize that a woman with a high body fat percentage, say at 40 percent, can eat such small amounts of food and still gain weight, while a woman with 20 percent body fat can eat way more food and stay at her ideal size. It doesn't seem fair.

But you can change the situation. Get that body fat down through strength training and use the "passive" activity of your higher metabolism to stay at your ideal size.

Maintain Your Ideal Size

We question whether a person can really lose weight through exercise alone. We actually have never seen this happen. We suppose that if a person went from being totally sedentary to running in marathons that he or she would lose weight. But we have never seen this happen.

We know that a person could conceivably gain weight from exercise. Since muscle weighs more than fat, a person could do strength training and gain weight, yet fit into his or her clothes better. In other words, the person could be a smaller size and yet weigh more. At that point, who cares? The person looks great.

But research shows over and over again that the people who maintain weight loss are the people who continue to exercise over their lifetime. This is because of the boost in metabolism and because exercise lifts mood, soothes anxiety, and improves health. When you feel good about yourself, you tend to make healthier decisions about food and eating.

Thinspiration

Sandy is a perfect example of being at her ideal size all her life. But as a result of getting older and letting her exercise regimen go by the wayside, she put on too many inches. As she says, "I am intelligent and teach others this concept—I live with a triathlete and marathoner for goodness sake! I feel better when I exercise, and I can go months doing regular exercise … but if I get out of the habit because of an extended vacation or whatever, it might take me months to get back into a regular routine again.

"It is just a matter of not being my top priority—I'd rather do other things. I am my best at exercise when I do it first thing in the morning and go to work a little later rather than trying to work it in after work. My early evenings are not consistent, and after supper I am surely not going to rev up my exercise motor! This whole subject is so interesting to me. The motivation has to come from within … and at first one just has to tell herself that it just won't be fun—but it has to be done—then it does become fun. I know to use a variety of exercise techniques so I don't get into a rut."

Shape Comes from Muscles

If you lost a lot of weight and did not exercise as you were losing it, you might get to your ideal size, but you could never get close to your desired shape.

Joan started at a size 22. Within a year and a half, she was wearing a size 8. This is terrific. She exercised by doing the five Tibetan exercises (see Chapter 17) every day, and she rode her exercise bike three times a week. She looked terrific as a size 8, and you couldn't tell that she had ever been overweight.

But if she hadn't exercised—oh, dear. Joan would have had sagging, loose skin all over her body. Her muscles would have been flabby. At that point, no amount of exercise could have firmed up the sagging, loose skin. Her only alternative would have been plastic surgery and lots of it.

Don't let this happen to you. If you exercise as you lose weight, your skin firms up and gets toned as you lose each ounce and pound. It sort of shrinkwraps to fit your muscles. But if you don't strengthen, stretch, and do cardio as you lose weight, the damage can be irreparable. We want you to look good in your clothes and on the beach. We want you to have your dream come true.

If you think you may need some nips and tucks after weight loss, make sure to maintain your weight loss for at least nine months before you opt for surgery. Yes, we have friends who had the work done too soon and then gained the weight back. It's not a good picture.

Goodbye, Blues

Aerobic exercise produces wonderful brain chemicals called endorphins. To get them in circulation, you need to break a sweat and do at least 20 minutes of aerobics or cardio exercise at a time. Less just isn't enough.

The flood of endorphins has been called the runner's high. They make you feel good. They lift your moods, even for hours after you are done exercising.

If you get the late-afternoon blues, if you fight anxiety and depression, get your endorphin lift regularly. If you are a stress eater, you can break the pattern by doing regular cardio workouts.

Our favorite story about the endorphin lift is about a woman who was so depressed she wanted to commit suicide. But, of course, she didn't want her family to suffer because of this, so she devised a plan to slowly kill herself. She would go out running so hard and so long that she would die. Well, she didn't die the first day, so she set out the second day, and the third, and the fourth. Soon she felt so good that she no longer wanted to die; in fact, she wanted to live. She cured her own deep depression through using those endorphins.

We find it easier to do the cardio when we remember and enjoy the day-to-day benefits of soothed anxiety and happier moods. This activity also forestalls lots of stress eating. Other activities that can soothe stress eating before it starts are found in Chapter 8.

Exercise Your Mental Function

Recent studies show that people who exercise think better. They score better on tests. They exhibit more creativity than when they don't exercise. Yes, exercise improves brain functioning.

Do you want your children to get better grades? Go shoot hoops after school with them. Ride bikes with them or take them with you to the gym.

Do you want to be more creative or to perform better at work? Get your regular dose of exercise and do it for life. Exercise increases cerebral blood flow and stimulates nerve cell growth.

Energy

If you feel sluggish and low on energy, by now you know the solution: get out and move. In earlier chapters, you garnered eating suggestions to correct late-afternoon tiredness. Now you know what else to do. Exercise every day or every other day and you will be amazed. You could look up at the clock and discover that you just sailed through the late afternoon and it's already time to quit work or eat dinner.

You will have energy to keep up with the kids or your spouse. You will have energy to enjoy social activities in the evening and not collapse after dinner in front of the TV— but perhaps not at first. As Sandy says, "When I haven't exercised regularly and I start up my exercise program again with aerobics in the mornings, I come in from my walk or finish my videotape and I am exhausted! I probably start back at the level where I left off a few months before, but I hate that feeling of tiredness rather than the energy I want!"

Overall, Your Health

The most significant activity to have good health throughout your life is to exercise. Nothing else counts as much as exercise. Food choices and supplements are important, but overall, nothing beats exercise for keeping you healthy.

It strengthens bones, eases hormonal difficulties, strengthens your heart, keeps blood pressure in a healthy range, and keeps your digestion and elimination functioning well. It even helps prevent certain forms of cancer.

What's not to like about exercise? Most likely, the fact that you have to do it. You have to make it a priority. Yes, we all have those days when we just don't want to do it. Taking a day off is fine. Taking two days off is risky. It is too easy to just stop exercising and blow it off.

Do whatever it takes to exercise. Do it with a friend, schedule it into your daily agenda, do it with a trainer or your spouse or children. Do it and the rewards will speak loudly.

Remember to get in motion. That is the best way to *stay* in motion.

The Least You Need to Know

◆ Exercise is essential for long-term weight maintenance.

◆ The inconveniences of exercise are insignificant compared to the enormous benefits.

◆ Exercise gives you the shape you want as you get to your ideal size, but it alone doesn't make you lose weight.

◆ Increasing muscle mass through strength training lowers your body fat content and boosts metabolism.

◆ The absolute best activity you can do for your overall health is to exercise regularly.

Chapter 16

The Essence of Exercise

In This Chapter

- ◆ What exercise does for you
- ◆ Easing into a good exercise routine
- ◆ Proper form matters
- ◆ Gaining health benefits
- ◆ Lightening your stress load

The essence of exercise is doing what your body was designed to do—use your muscles. Using your muscles is primitive. It's refreshing. It makes you feel good. It keeps you healthy. And regular exercise is a significant factor to help you keep excess weight off for life.

Yes, some thin people do not exercise regularly. Are you one of them? Probably not. Can you claim any benefits to your health and weight loss from *not* exercising? Of course not. Let exercise become as routine and important to you as brushing your teeth. You wouldn't think of not brushing your teeth. Make it so that you wouldn't think of not exercising every day or every other day. It's that important.

Exercise Is Your Friend

Exercise is my friend? No way! Okay, we'll grant that most friends don't make you sweat, but you should get on good terms with exercise if you want to lose weight and keep it off. It works!

Regular exercise, if it includes both strength and cardio training, will boost your metabolic rate and help you burn fat faster. Recent studies show that subjects who didn't exercise had a reduced capacity to burn stored fat, both during exercise and when at rest. With regular exercise, you even burn more fuel when you sleep than if you are sedentary.

Thinspiration

Start affirming your commitment to exercise … even as you read this chapter. Don't give in to the negative self-talk that produces innumerable excuses for why you didn't or can't exercise. A positive attitude has helped countless individuals who were couch potatoes become fit for life. You *can* do it!

You can lose weight without exercising, but it will be harder to do, and you won't feel as energized. We're not talking about becoming a marathoner or gym-aholic. We want you to develop an exercise program that fits you, your body, and your lifestyle.

Even low-intensity exercise, such as walking three times a week, is adequate to prevent the post weight-loss decline in the rate of fat burning. This represents the minimal amount of exercise you need to do. However, it's best to do cardio and strength training plus flexibility work because the health and fat-loss benefits are even more enticing.

What Doesn't Count as Exercise

Some forms of recreation just aren't going to give you good results for fat burning, an increase in metabolism, and overall excellent health. Some people may want to think these are exercise, but they simply don't count. There are the obvious ones: billiards, television, video games, bridge, poker, and miniature golf, to name a few. Also, don't expect much exercise benefit from bowling, horseshoes, golfing with a cart, hitting balls at the driving range, or fishing.

Weighty Warning

Watching an exercise video while sitting on the sofa doesn't count as exercise, and we doubt it will "inspire" you to exercise later. When you pop an exercise video into the VCR, be ready to work out with the instructor.

None of these activities count as exercise, but they can be fun and certainly are recreational. Enjoy them if you're so inclined, but you'll also need to have a real exercise plan.

Starting to Exercise

The hardest part about starting a personal exercise program is often just that—starting. For many of us, it's pretty intimidating. We become more self-conscious of our bodies and fear that we'll somehow "fail" at exercising. Your body is designed for motion and exercise. You'll do fine. To help you get off on the right foot, so to speak, the next few sections cover some things to consider.

Start Slow to Win the Race

If you start out at a level that is too tough for you, you may experience lots of pain and virtually no gain. Be sure to honor the current state of your body and your fitness level before you dive in. If you're out of shape, build up your strength and stamina. Remember that you're into exercise for the long haul, in essence for the rest of your life. You can afford the time it takes to get your body into shape. When a person goes too fast, the ensuing bodily aches and pains can prevent further exercise ... and destroy motivation. Don't let this happen!

Remember the race between the tortoise and the hare? The tortoise started slow but eventually won the race. When it comes to exercising, you can start slow and build up your "speed" over time to win your personal challenge. You don't need to compete with anyone!

Thinspiration

By tuning in to the wisdom you have in your body already, you can learn how to exercise to suit your personal needs. Just as you have learned how to eat based on your body's signals, so, too, can you learn how to exercise by listening to your body's wisdom.

Clothing to Sweat In

Wear clothing appropriate to the type of exercise you're doing. Go for comfort and practicality. Some forms of exercise require more fitted leotards and tights. Some are fine with loose-fitting T-shirts and gym shorts. Forget how you look in exercise clothes and go for practicality and comfort. You're going to look better day after day.

You don't need to think that you are supposed to compete with all the beautiful and buff bodies at the gym. You are there to take care of yourself, just as they are. Wear what works and what feels comfortable.

Remember the Sunscreen

Exercises done outdoors—biking, hiking, running, walking, and so on—are a double treat for many of us because we get the added benefits of sunshine and fresh air. But

Weighty Warning

Skin cancer has become one of the most prevalent forms of cancer in the United States. If you exercise outside, wear appropriate clothing and use sunscreen to protect your skin.

do use sunscreen. Your skin isn't designed to be cooked, not even browned! Skin cancer is a serious problem these days, and it isn't selective. It will attack the skin of a buff athlete as quickly as anyone else.

Pain Isn't Required

Forget the famous exercise motto of "no pain, no gain." It's great for jocks, jockettes, and gym junkies. At the beginning, just do the exercises and avoid the pain. Right now, you are easing into a life-long exercise program.

Always listen to your body for when it is time to stop an exercise and when it is time to push harder. This will prevent overdoing it and also underdoing it. In some exercise classes, instructors keep yelling for you to "Push it!" or "Go harder!" Unless you like being provoked like that, either ignore the instructor and listen to your body or find another class. It's absolutely not essential for you to overexert yourself to the point of being exhausted or sore.

Many elegant exercise choices available today produce terrific strength and tone with virtually no pain. We tell all in the next chapter.

Body of Knowledge

An exercise physiologist can suggest alternative modification methods for different exercises to compensate for any medical or bodily conditions you have.

Doctor's Checkup

It's always a good idea to check with your doctor before you begin an exercise program, especially if you have a particular health concern such as a heart condition or a bad back. However, doctors today almost universally encourage regular exercise. If you plan to engage the services of a personal trainer, work out in a class, or exercise with a group, make sure the group leader knows of any physical limitations you may have.

An Intelligent Exercise Approach

Some self-discipline and common sense will go a long way toward making exercise effective for you. Remember that this is your exercise program; you're not in a military boot camp. If you have a limited range of motion, only go as far as you're comfortable with each exercise. It's tempting to try to keep up or even compete in group classes, but you don't need to do this. In fact, you shouldn't. Instead, listen to your body and do only what you can do. Ask the instructor's advice when necessary.

At one time, Mimi engaged the services of a personal trainer who came to her home three times a week. Even though she has a weak rotator cuff in her right shoulder, the trainer kept demanding that she work the shoulder in a way that was painful. He ignored her discomfort. What an insensitive lout! Later, her doctor explained that some people of northern European descent (such as herself) naturally had this condition, and surgery wasn't a good solution. His suggestion: Do as much exercise as possible and stop short of the pain.

Fortunately, most knowledgeable personal trainers won't make the same mistake. Be sure to check credentials and references if you engage the services of a personal trainer. If you have an injury or a specific muscle weakness, ask the trainer to show you how to strengthen the area or how to get the same results without further injuring yourself.

> **CAUTION**
>
> **Weighty Warning**
>
> Your exercise program should be pain free. If any part of your body hurts, stop immediately. Push yourself enough to get a good workout but not so far that you get injured. Injuries ruin your momentum and require time for recovery.

Darlene was enticed into a very intense weight-training program through the startling before and after pictures in the newspaper. The program was advertised as only one hour a week to attaining the perfect body. But, oh boy, what an hour it proved to be! In class one evening, Darlene was doing sit-ups with over 40 pounds of weights—buckshot sewed into bags—resting on her stomach and midriff. Hard? You bet! She popped a rib out of place! Yes, the ambulance came.

You don't need to go to extremes to get fit, nor should you ever hurt yourself. Take it easy and reach your goal like the tortoise rather than the hare.

Spot Reducing

Spot reducing works ... at times. If you have a puffy tummy and want to streamline it, you can. Spot reducing doesn't necessarily mean losing weight at one specific part of your body. It means tightening up or elongating certain muscle groups. Spot reducing needs to be part of a complete whole-body exercise program.

> **Body of Knowledge**
>
> Spot reducing can help when your body is ready for it. It's actually hard to tell what body areas require special attention until you get close to your ideal size. Many things will change about your body as you lose weight and exercise, so be patient and don't focus on spot reducing.

Stacy was about 5'1" and wanted to trim her thighs. She got on the Stairmaster day after day, trying to whip those thighs into shape. And her hard work did produce a new shape—bigger thighs!

Why? Because her body shape and musculature was such that she had short thigh-bones. As she stepped and stepped, her thighs got stronger and stronger, packing on more and more muscle. On her small body, her thighs got bigger, the opposite of her goal! Rather than elongating the muscles, she was bulking them up. A better choice for her would have been exercises that elongated her thigh muscles, such as yoga, Pilates, and stretching.

If you are now overweight, spot reducing won't have much value until you get closer to your ideal size and can actually see what you want to elongate and what you want to firm up. Be patient, that day will come.

Push Beyond Your Limits

Part of the "game" of exercise is to gradually and continually push your body's limits. If right now your limit is running a half-mile, eventually you will be able to double that. Don't think of this as a competition or even that more is better. Just know that in a couple months, you'll want to do more because your body will be ready to do more.

Thinspiration

Keep on keeping on. The more you get into the flow of regular exercise, the more you will love doing it. The health and weight-loss benefits begin the minute you start your program, and they grow as you continue your program. Be prepared to keep getting better, stronger, and more in control of your body and your weight.

Moving Beyond Mere Movement

Don't confuse exercise with movement. Movement is better than being sedentary, but you'll need other kinds of exercise, too. Movement includes simple activities such as walking, climbing a few flights of stairs instead of the taking the elevator, or parking at the far end of a parking lot and walking the extra steps to the grocery store. These kinds of activities are low intensity, however, and don't increase your pulse rate enough to release endorphins, nor to build muscle mass, nor to make a significant reduction in body fat.

Lean Lingo

Clickers and pedometers are small devices that attach to one's waistband or belt. They measure how many steps a person takes. A common goal is to take 10,000 steps a day, which is equivalent to walking about 4 to 5 miles.

Activities such as walking are sure better for you than sitting around. Often people measure movement with *clickers* or *pedometers*. These register how many steps you take—in other words, how much you're moving. Studies show that on average, 10,000 clicks or steps a day will reduce blood pressure and lower cholesterol. Moving your body will make you stronger and will burn calories. Wearing a pedometer is like having a personal trainer on your hip, counting your results and silently urging you to move more.

Unfortunately, low-intensity movement exercises don't produce the same fat-burning benefits as a higher-intensity workout. Plus, a high-intensity workout boosts your metabolism and keeps it high for a while after your workout. To get the best shape, tone, and cardio benefits from exercise, you'll need to do more than move, but what a great way to start. As you progress, increase the cardio intensity and add in strength training and flexibility exercises regularly to have a complete workout.

Do Them Correctly

You'll be amazed at the extra benefits you'll get when you perform exercises correctly. It really does make a difference, and you don't want to waste one moment doing an exercise incorrectly. Learn the correct posture for using everything from your stationary exercise bike to weight-lifting equipment.

Do you have any idea how many times we've seen people spend hours on stair-stepping machine, slumped over the hand rails as if they need them to keep from keeling over. They may be doing some good, but they sure aren't getting the full benefit of the exercise. You can learn proper techniques from a trainer, a video, or a book. Get your form down right!

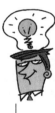

Thinspiration

Correct posture makes a big difference. If you're going to exercise at all, you may as well do it correctly.

Exercise and Your Health

The single most significant factor in improving one's health is exercise. Research strongly indicates that exercise alone can improve your health, decrease the risk of serious illness, and reverse some of the degenerative effects of aging. Here's what exercise does for you:

◆ **Strengthens your heart.** The heart is a muscle, and it benefits from regular cardiovascular exercise. This means aerobics that will boost your heart rate. A stronger heart can avert arteriosclerosis and reduce high cholesterol and high blood pressure.

◆ **Increases lung capacity.** Exercise allows your lungs to increase their capacity to hold more oxygen. Exercise also lets your body utilize the oxygen it gets more efficiently, which increases your metabolism.

♦ **Increases bone density.** A woman who performs weight-bearing exercises regularly can increase her bone density and prevent the onset of osteoporosis. Studies show that even elderly women can benefit from weight-bearing exercise.

♦ **Improves insulin utilization.** Regular exercise lets your body reduce high levels of insulin. High levels can lead to storing more fat and to type 2 diabetes.

♦ **Helps prevent certain kinds of cancers.** Yes, you can reduce your risk of certain kinds of cancer, such as colorectal cancer, by engaging in regular exercise.

♦ **Reduces the effects of aging.** Exercise improves muscle tone and counteracts the decrease in metabolic rate that usually comes with age.

♦ **Lessens depression and anxiety.** The release of endorphins that occurs after about 20 minutes of cardiovascular or aerobic exercise can lift one's mood for a couple of hours, perhaps even days. The endorphins soothe anxiety and reduce depression.

♦ **Increases mental acuity.** Studies indicate that people who exercise regularly have better mental alertness and prowess than those who don't.

Thinspiration

Instead of eating to tackle stress, work up a sweat. The endorphins released from 20 minutes of vigorous exercise can help you say goodbye forever to stress eating.

♦ **Helps balance hormones.** Hormones are responsible for energy, sex drive, moods, digestion, and many other bodily functions. Having balanced hormones can reduce the effects of aging and boost your energy.

The health benefits of regular exercise will let you enjoy living at your ideal size. We especially like that endorphin-stimulating exercise can reduce depression and lessen anxiety.

The Least You Need to Know

♦ People who maintain weight loss the best are those who exercise regularly.

♦ Start your exercise program slowly and work up gradually to optimum exercise levels.

♦ The health benefits of exercise are significant, contribute to overall well-being, and reduce the effects of aging.

♦ Regular exercise will help you reduce the anxiety that often brings on overeating.

Chapter 17

Variety Is the Spice of Exercise

In This Chapter

- ◆ The three basic types of exercise
- ◆ The great variety of exercise choices
- ◆ Choosing exercises wisely
- ◆ Exercise can be fun
- ◆ The fabulous five Tibetans

There are three health-related fitness components you should include in your exercise program: a cardio-respiratory component (aerobic/cardio), a muscle strength and endurance component (strength training), and a flexibility component (stretching).

Yes, you need to have all three activities in your exercise program (including warm-up and cool-down). Why? Because you deserve all the wonderful results. Here's the good news: Many exercises encompass all three areas, and we'll show you which ones.

Aerobic/Cardio Exercise

Over the past 20 years the term "cardio" has gradually replaced the term "aerobic," but in this chapter we're going to use them almost interchangeably. The basic premise is simple: You should exercise enough to speed up your heart rate and keep it up for at least 20 minutes. Why 20 minutes? Because it takes at least that long for your heart to work hard enough for you to experience the cardiovascular and endorphin benefits.

That's right, get your heart rate up and keep it up for at least 20 minutes per session, ideally daily. Huff and puff a little. Break out in a sweat. Burn energy. Move fast. Vigorous exercise for 45 minutes every other day is a good alternative.

Cardio builds your endurance, strengthens your heart, and increases your lung capacity. It releases endorphins, those wonderful mood-elevating brain chemicals. Exercise is one time when harnessing the power of drugs is fine because your body is making them. They're legal, they're free, and in fact, they're a natural high that your body is meant to enjoy.

Thinspiration

The amount of recommended exercise can sound intimidating at first. Don't let it stop you. Start your exercise program slowly and work up to the recommended amount. No matter what shape you are in now, within a couple months, you will be delighted with your progress. Stay with it.

You've got a lot of choices for the cardio/aerobic part of your workout. Choose one or more that you can do every day or every other day. They don't need to be fancy or elaborate. If you have a stationary bike, just schedule yourself to start peddling. Your simple goal is to elevate your heart rate for 20 minutes or more. Many clubs have the television blaring as people sweat on the various cardio machines. Some people read. But whatever you do, get your cardio exercise.

Here are target heart rates based on your age. Choose the age closest to yours. Try to keep your heart rate between the minimum and maximum for the duration of your cardio workout.

Age	Minimum	Moderate	Maximum
20	125	145	165
30	120	138	155
40	115	130	145
50	110	125	140
60	105	118	130
70	95	110	125
80	90	103	115

Measure your heart rate this way: Count your pulse by touching your fingers to the opposite wrist or to the pulse point in your neck. Count beats for 6 seconds. Multiply by 10 and that is your heart rate. If your heart rate stays close to the minimum target range for your age, increase your exercise session beyond 20 minutes or pick up the pace.

Here are some super choices for cardio/aerobic exercise:

◆ **Biking.** Bike either outdoors on a street bike or mountain bike or indoors on a stationary bike. It's terrific for low-stress, high-intensity aerobic fitness. Your only cost is the cost of your equipment—a stationary bike or one that moves.

◆ **Classes.** There's a vast variety of aerobic fitness classes: step classes, aerobic dancing classes, spinning classes, and classes like Jazzercise. Classes are widely available at health clubs, studios, and local recreation centers.

◆ **Cardio equipment.** These include treadmills, cross-country-skiing machines, elliptical trainers, stepping machines, and rowing machines. Most health and fitness facilities offer all these and more. Find the ones you like the best and start moving. Many motels and hotels offer an exercise room with equipment, so you can get your exercise easily when you travel.

◆ **Cardio/aerobic videotapes.** There are hundreds of good routines available on video and DVD. Videos let you exercise at home without having to go out and can save you time. See Appendix B for sources of videos.

◆ **Swimming.** Swimming is great exercise, either indoors or outdoors, and indoor pools make swimming a year-round option. The expense involved is a health club or pool membership. Swimming also elongates muscles; we like that.

◆ **Walking.** Plain old walking can count as cardio/aerobic exercise if you can get your heart rate up. But to do that, a casual stroll won't help. You've got to walk *fast*. We have friends who walk outdoors in good weather and who walk in shopping malls when it's raining or snowing. Some walkers enhance their workout by wearing shoes with weighted soles. These improve muscle tone in the lower body and increase the amount of physical energy expended. Sandy wears weighted shoes during work hours at the hospital. She

Weighty Warning

Think carefully before you invest in expensive exercise equipment for your home. How often will you use it? Will you stick with it for years? If you're purchasing home exercise equipment with the hope that spending that much money will motivate you to use it, your plan is flawed and you could find your equipment gathering dust.

Thinspiration

Walking is excellent at the beginning of your exercise program. As you progress, however, we urge you to add in more strenuous exercise that gives you more cardio/aerobic benefit and that releases those uplifting endorphins. Walking won't give you that lift. That's why it's called the "runner's high," not the "walker's high!"

finds them a great way to intensify her walking throughout the day. Plus she enjoys the lower-body firming from wearing them. (See Appendix B for more information on weighted shoes.) Avoid using ankle weights when you walk or climb stairs. They put too much stress on the ankle and knee joints and can cause harm.

◆ **Jogging, running, and race walking.** Purchase a good pair of shoes and go enjoy the outdoors. Unlike noisy gym classes, these activities give you an opportunity to take in beautiful scenery and off-street trails as you raise your heart rate.

◆ **Rebounding using a mini trampoline or rebounder boots.** These give you a bouncing effect—kind of like bouncing on a pogo stick. Rebounding gets your endorphins flowing faster than many other forms of cardio/aerobic exercise, and it feels great. Some research shows that rebounding can be detoxifying for the body (great!) because it may stimulate the flow of lymph fluid. We like the rebounding boots for both jogging outside and doing aerobic dancing indoors. You can find more info on rebounding boots in Appendix B.

Rebounder boots are great for cardio exercise that gets your endorphins energized.

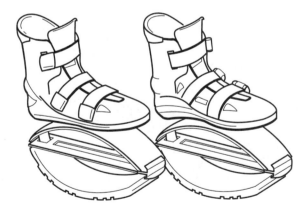

Strength Training—Get Strong

Strength training! But I don't want to look like Arnold Schwarzenegger! Good. Because that's not what we're talking about. Basic strength training is designed to increase your muscle tone, give your muscles shape and strength, and increase your metabolic rate. It will alter your body composition from flabby fat to calorie-gobbling muscles and will make weight control much, much easier.

Strength training is also excellent for keeping your bones strong and avoiding osteoporosis, for reducing your body fat percentage, and for boosting your metabolism.

Today, there are many excellent exercise choices for strength training. It used to be that the only viable choice was using free weights or weight-training machines. They have stood the test of time. Today, however, there are other alternatives that work equally well. We know of several women who have reduced their body fat percentage by 10 points—say from 28 percent to 18 percent, or from 38 percent to 28 percent—just by doing core conditioning (also known as Pilates-type exercises) in one-hour sessions, two times a week, for six months.

Strength training can turn upper arms from flabby into sexy. Ditto backs, thighs, and tummies. It can improve posture. The key to building terrific muscles is to keep upping the intensity of your workout over time. Gradually increase the weight and the resistance as you get stronger. For example, when two- or three-pound weights get easy for your arm exercises, it's time to use five-pound weights.

Here's a quick look at several forms of strength training. Find one or two that you enjoy and can do at least two times a week. You don't need to do them daily. Each of these choices offers different benefits, but when doing strength training, make sure to include exercises for your whole body. Work every muscle group. Also, be attentive to form and breathing because proper technique makes a big difference in your overall results.

> **Body of Knowledge**
>
> Strength training uses weights and resistance to put greater than normal stress on your muscles. (Just imagine lifting a dumbbell.) Under this strain, you create tiny, harmless tears in the muscle fibers. When you rest for a day or so between strength training sessions, the muscles heal, resulting in stronger and more clearly defined muscles.

> **Thinspiration**
>
> You can miss a week or two of strength training, but it will begin to show quickly in how your clothes fit … or don't. Thank goodness that when you restart your program, the results return quickly.

- ◆ **Free weights.** Barbells and dumbbells are great for developing your major muscles and may be used to create bulk. The number of repetitions and the speed of repetitions will affect the results you get. It's essential that you use free weights in the correct alignment; otherwise, your efforts will be wasted. Learn how before you embark on free-weights training. You can learn from an instructor, a book, or a video. You can use free weights at the gym and also set up a home program. A new form of weight lifting is called "super slow". Slowing down the speed of each repetition makes the muscles work harder and more precisely. Using free weights doesn't develop flexibility or elongate muscles, so be sure you add flexibility exercises to your program.

♦ **Weight-training machines.** These are available in most health clubs. The machines work major muscles and are easy to use because they help ensure proper alignment. You can also purchase these machines for your home. Keep in mind that these machines don't increase flexibility or lengthen muscles.

♦ **Core conditioning or Pilates.** These exercises can be done in a studio or class with an instructor or at home with videos or a book. They emphasize careful and precise movements to strengthen the body's core muscles in the abdomen area. All of the exercises, even for arms and legs, are done with a focus on using the abdominal muscles for stability. Pilates programs work all the muscles: the major muscles and the smaller muscles. A big plus is that Pilates develops strength, elongated muscles, and flexibility. For many, it helps improve posture. A side benefit: It's highly relaxing.

Body of Knowledge

A highly effective and efficient way to do strength training is what's known as Super Slow. Using this technique, you slow down your movements so that it takes two, three, or four times longer to do each repetition. Advocates say muscles get more of a workout because they're working constantly and don't get an easier ride because of the momentum of more rapid repetitions. The Super Slow approach works for almost all types of strength training.

♦ **Yoga.** Yoga creates balance, strength, and flexibility. It can be done in class or at home with a video or book. Yoga originated in India thousands of years ago to promote health and well-being. Yoga sometimes looks easy, but it isn't. It requires attentiveness and accurate alignment. Yoga is an excellent choice, especially if you haven't been exercising recently. It lets you create balance, strength, and flexibility in the highly accepting and nurturing environment of a yoga studio or, of course, your own home.

♦ **Fitness ball.** These large balls, which range from 45 cm to 75 cm in diameter, promote strength and balance plus stretching. The exercises look simple, but the extra challenge is that you need to balance while doing those sit-ups and leg extensions. One of the hardest workouts we've ever had was on a ball. They come with a nifty small air pump, so you can take the ball when you travel. The balls cost in the range of $30 to $40. There are excellent videos for the fitness ball that range from easy and slow to highly challenging. We keep aspiring to be able to perform all the exercises on these videos. Some videos for the fitness ball are great for aerobic/cardio conditioning. Fitness ball classes are also offered at many health clubs.

Thinspiration

Strength-building exercises deliver quick visible results. As you continue to build muscle strength, the results only get better. Within six months of two sessions a week, you'll enjoy how your clothes look on you and how you feel.

◆ **Fitness circle.** This piece of equipment has a $1^{1}/_{4}$-inch band of steel wrapped three times to form a circle, or ring, about 18 inches in diameter plus handles. You use the circle for resistance, such as doing a very slow sit-up while squeezing it between your knees. By using any one of the many videos or DVDs available on the fitness circle, you can have a complete and comprehensive strength and stretching session in 30 minutes. It can be packed in a suitcase. Cost varies from $20 on up, but the $20 version works well.

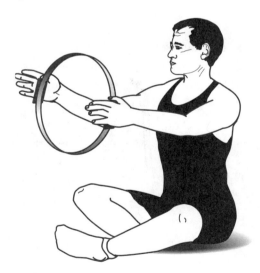

The fitness circle lets you gain stronger muscles as you do Pilates mat exercises.

The fitness ball, flex band, and fitness circle are equipment used in Pilates workouts. Check out Appendix B for information on where to purchase videos for this equipment. If you like using this list of simple equipment and you really fall in love with the elegant Pilates exercise system, you can go full out and purchase the Pilates Reformer.

Thinspiration

Check out Pilates-based exercises. Pilates, based on strength and flexibility techniques that Joseph Pilates taught to classical dancers beginning in the 1930s, is the hottest exercise approach sweeping the country. We predict it will be here long after other fads have passed on. The results you'll enjoy are most likely in line with how you want to look: strong, long, lean muscles and better posture. Many people even say they've gotten taller from doing Pilates! Find out for yourself. Check out your local phone book or health clubs near you for a beginner class or lesson.

All Pilates strength-building exercises require you to participate actively—by focusing on your body and concentrating on your form. This has a way of making Pilates very relaxing because it's impossible to worry about or even think about much else when you're doing it. The intense focus actually assists you in getting the full benefit from Pilates exercises. An added plus is that you don't sweat much but you still get the strength and flexibility results you want.

Flexibility

Can you easily bend over to touch your toes? Can you sit cross-legged on the floor? If not, your body needs more flexibility. A flexible body is such a treat. It gives your movements grace and fluidity. It makes you look great. It keeps your spine strong and reduces the risk of injury.

Thinspiration

Stretching is almost guaranteed to make you feel better, and you don't need to naturally be a human pretzel to enjoy it. If you're out of shape, stretching exercises will pay off right away. You'll learn to feel how your body works, will begin to elongate your muscles, and will feel more relaxed.

You gain flexibility from stretching exercises that elongate the body muscles. Stretching feels good. It's typically relaxing because, as you stretch, you release the tension held in your muscles.

We need to talk for a moment here about your tummy. If you're finding that all the abdominal crunches in the world aren't giving you a flat tummy, try stretching. Do a slow backbend over a fitness ball, stretching each part of the front of the body as you slowly roll back over the ball. Then turn over face down and stretch your back. This elongates your abdominal muscles and feels great.

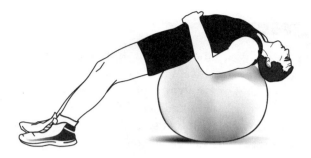

Recline over the FitBall for an excellent abdominal stretch.

Here are some forms of exercise that will help you stretch:

- Pilates

- Yoga

- Tibetans

- Flexibility and stretching classes

- Stretching videos and books

We suggest that you also stretch after your cardio workouts and after strength training. In fact, stretch every day just for the utter joy of it.

Combination Programs

There are several ways to combine more than one type of exercise at the same time. Dancing, karate, Tae Bo, and martial arts offer you various combinations of cardio/ aerobic, flexibility, and strength training. If you want to take up one of these activities, what better time than now?

Thinspiration

Lucy's hiking for recreation: "As my body adapted to mountain hiking, I experienced hiking as the perfect date with my husband. We now either hike or snow shoe most weekends. We pack along books on wildflowers and birds. We love being out in the clear air. And we especially enjoy doing it together. Hiking is so utterly exhilarating. It feels good all over."

Sandy's dancing classes for recreation: "My husband and I take weekly dance classes as a way to handle being empty nesters. Now we have a regular dance 'date' every week and enjoy the movement and fun together. Nothing gets in the way of our dance date."

Get Out and Recreate

Cardio, strength, and flexibility are the basics for exercise, but let's not get too serious and forget that there are lots of great ways to exercise when you're also having fun. So recreate, okay? Find a friend or family member who would enjoy doing recreational activities with you. Couples and families that enjoy recreational exercise together are healthier and do a better job of staying at their ideal size. Here's a partial list of recreational activities that feature great exercise:

- Dancing or dance lessons
- Tennis
- Racquetball
- Squash
- Soccer
- Hiking
- Biking
- Kayaking
- Running races
- Walkathons
- Snow shoeing
- Skiing
- Cross-country skiing

A Daily Dose of Five Essential Exercises

Years ago, in 1939, a small book titled *Ancient Secret of the Fountain of Youth* was published. Written by Peter Keldor, it told the story of an aging colonel who went to Tibet and returned 10 years later, looking many years younger. The colonel attributed his youthful appearance to doing these five exercises every day. They're affectionately known as the Tibetans.

The Tibetans get your heart pumping, although not long enough for full cardio benefits. They strengthen your muscles and improve your flexibility. Even better, they give you a great lift, like you had a cup of coffee without the coffee.

The five Tibetans have been passed around quietly for years, and those of us who do them routinely would never stop. Why? Because they deliver. After you've done the five Tibetan exercises for about three months, you'll notice you no longer have a double chin. It has vanished. Women eventually discover that their midriffs are sort of slinkier, and men often have lost several belt sizes … even without losing weight.

The reported benefits of the Tibetans are as follows:

- Double chin gone
- Midriff slimmer
- Upper arms firmer
- More energy
- Increased muscle tone
- Early morning wake-up lift

Thinspiration

On my forty-fifth birthday, I, Lucy, received a copy of the *Ancient Secrets of the Fountain of Youth* from my 19-year-old son. He gave me the book because, as he said, "Mom, you're getting old." Since that time, I have done the five simple Tibetan exercises faithfully every morning as I start my day. In just 5 to 10 minutes, I'm ready to take on whatever the day brings.

The following is what researchers say the five Tibetans do for the body:

- Stimulate the reticular activating system of the brain.
- Balance the right and left hemispheres of the brain, which means you think more clearly. (You should definitely do the Tibetans before an exam or an important presentation!)
- Balance the body's hormonal system.
- Strengthen bones, as the exercises are weight bearing.
- Improve the body's immune system.
- Build muscle strength.
- Reduce body fat percentage.
- Boost metabolism.
- Align and strengthen the spine, plus make it more supple.
- Lighten menopausal symptoms.
- Lessen premenstrual symptoms.
- Help relieve the discomfort of arthritis and other aches and pains.

While Joe was on an extended business trip to London, he began doing the Tibetans two times a day, morning and late afternoon. He was careful to eat an amount of food the size of his fist three times a day. Plus he walked a lot. By the time he returned home to Australia, Joe had lost 4 inches around his waist. His wife didn't recognize him when he appeared at the front door. Joe was 56 years old.

Doing the Tibetans

We recommend that you do the Tibetans every morning when you wake up. They're easiest to do on an empty stomach. If the exercises seem too strenuous at first, refer to the book *Ancient Secrets of the Fountain of Youth, Part 2*, published by Doubleday, for starter exercises so that you can slowly build up strength to do the full recommended set.

For beginners, just start with three or four repetitions of each exercise for the first week. Then increase the number of repetitions by a few every week until you reach the full 21 repetitions. Do the repetitions of each exercise before moving on to the next exercise. If you never work all the way up to 21 each, don't worry; they will still deliver results.

The five Tibetan exercises can be performed anytime and virtually anywhere. It isn't necessary to do each exercise more than 21 times to receive all their benefits.

The Tibetans

Exercise 1: Standing with arms extended outward to the sides at shoulder height, spin your body toward your right hand. Go slowly at first and be sure to stop if you feel dizzy. Should you get dizzy, pick a spot on the wall and look at it until you feel clear headed. Eventually, you will be able to spin quickly without getting dizzy. In the beginning, just spin three complete rotations, eventually working up to 21.

Spinning seems like an odd exercise, and in a way it is. But it wakes your body up and seems to stimulate proper hormonal balance. There's a reason why children love to spin—because it feels good and it's good for you.

Exercise 2: First lie flat on the floor, face up. Fully extend your arms along your sides and place the palms of your hands against the floor, keeping the fingers close together. If you want, place your hands under your hips to brace your movement. Then raise your head off the floor, tucking the chin against the chest. As you do this, lift your legs, knees straight, into a vertical position, perpendicular to the floor. If possible, let the legs extend back over the body toward the head, but do not let the knees bend. Then slowly lower both your head and legs, knees straight, to the floor. Breathe in deeply as you lift your legs and breathe out as you lower your legs.

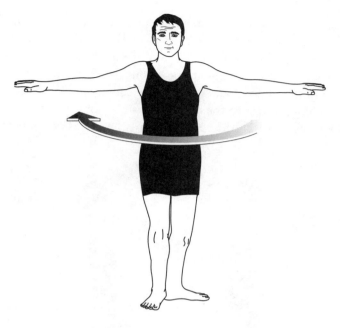

Exercise 1.

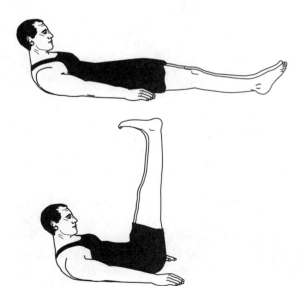

Exercise 2.

Exercise 3: Kneel on the floor with the torso of your body erect. Place your hands behind your back either in the middle back or lower back. Bend your neck and head forward, tucking the chin against the chest. Then move the head and neck backward slowly, arching your spine. As you arch, you brace your hands against your body for support. Go backward until you are looking up at the ceiling and your neck feels fully stretched. After the arching, return to the original position and start the second repetition. Breathe in deeply as you arch the spine and breathe out as you return to an erect position.

Exercise 3.

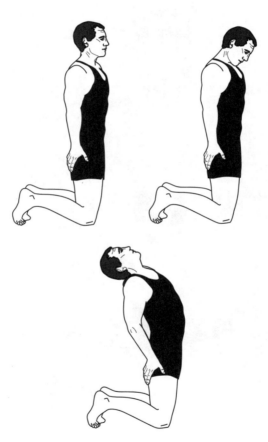

Exercise 4: Sit down on the floor with your legs straight out in front of you and your feet about 12 inches apart. Sit up straight and place the palms of your hands on the floor alongside your buttocks, fingers pointed toward your toes. Tuck your chin forward against the chest. Then slowly drop your head backward as far as it will go. At the same time, raise your body so that the knees bend while the arms remain straight.

The only body parts touching the floor are the palms of your hands and the soles of your feet.

The trunk of your body will be aligned with the upper legs, horizontal to the floor. Your body will be in the shape of a bench. Then tense every muscle in the body. Finally, relax your muscles as you return to the original sitting position and rest before repeating the procedure. Breathe in as you raise up, hold your breath as you tense the muscles, and breathe out completely as you come down.

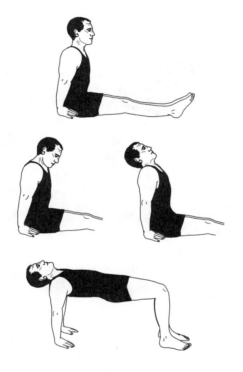

Exercise 4.

Exercise 5: When you perform the fifth exercise, your body is facing the floor with just your toes and hands on the floor. Make a tent shape out of your body, with your head tucked between your arms and your bottom up. Then move your torso toward the floor so that you are flexing the spine in reverse and look up at the ceiling. Breathe in deeply as you raise your body and breathe out fully as you lower it.

Exercise 5.

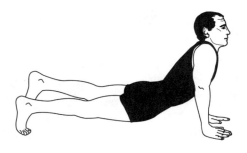

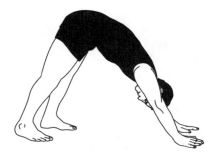

The five Tibetans are an exercise "extra" to boost your fitness progress. They're a great way to start the day, and they fit nicely with other parts of your exercise program. Clients rave about the results they get. You'll love the results, too.

The Least You Need to Know

- There are three kinds of exercise—aerobic/cardio, strength training, and stretching—that you should do to feel good, look good, and reach your ideal size.

- Choose the exercise approaches you like the best and that work for you and your family.

- Include regular recreational exercise for fun, variety, and the joy of the activity.

- Do the five Tibetans every day upon waking; they feel good and do great things for you and your body.

Chapter 18

Design Your Personal Exercise Plan

In This Chapter

- ◆ Choosing a personal exercise approach
- ◆ Setting exercise goals
- ◆ Overcoming exercise obstacles
- ◆ Keeping yourself motivated

By now you may be thinking, "How do I get all this exercise done and still have a life?" Or you may be wondering if the trick to weight loss is to exercise so much that you don't even have time to eat!

In this chapter, we'll show you how to design a program that works for you and that you can use with confidence. We want you to truly enjoy exercising, so it's important to figure out an approach that's just right for you.

Your Comfort Zone

The first thing you need to figure out is where you want to exercise. You'll want to feel comfortable about your selected place. You basically have three choices for day-in, day-out exercise: home, the *gym*, or both. You need to figure out which suits your lifestyle best and helps you stay on track. There are advantages and disadvantages to each.

Lean Lingo

Think of a **gym** as any place designed for exercise, such as a health club, a fitness center, a specialty studio, or a local recreational center. If you haven't been in a health club recently, you may be surprised by the range of equipment and classes available. You'll discover sophisticated exercise equipment, tennis or racquet courts, personal trainers, aerobic classes, Pilates instruction, yoga classes, and many other exercise offerings.

Benefits of at-home exercising:

◆ It may be more convenient for your schedule.

◆ You don't need to get dressed up.

◆ The shower is readily available.

◆ You don't need to drive anywhere.

◆ Instruction is available through excellent videos available today.

◆ You can hire a personal trainer to come to your home.

◆ You can use television or Internet exercise programs.

◆ It's efficient because you don't have travel time.

Drawbacks of at-home exercising:

◆ It requires lots of self-discipline.

◆ You are subject to distractions and interruptions from family members and the phone.

◆ Is not social. (This can be either good or bad depending on your preference.)

◆ It may require you to purchase equipment.

◆ It requires floor space to exercise.

Benefits of exercising at a gym:

◆ Professional, varied classes and groups.

◆ The opportunity to meet other people.

- Group motivation.

- Professional-quality exercise equipment.

- Encouragement to push yourself harder.

- Extra motivation because you are paying for it.

- Often offer courts for racquetball or tennis.

- May have swimming pool with lanes for aerobic swimmers.

- Personal trainers on hand for consultations.

Drawbacks of exercising at a gym:

- The hassle of getting there via car or other transportation.

- You may need to adapt your schedule to their classes.

- The monthly cost needs to be factored into your household budget.

- The possible awkwardness exercising in public.

- Nonprivate locker rooms.

Even if you join a gym, it's important to have a backup plan for exercising at home. Use it when you can't get to the gym or when you're traveling or on vacation. Yes, you hear us correctly. Just because you can't get to the gym is absolutely no excuse for missing your personal exercise appointment with yourself.

The Exercise Appointment

Do you use some form of calendar or appointment book? Or do you just keep a schedule in your head? In either case, make a date to exercise. At the beginning of every week, schedule your exercise appointments into your daily planner. Give yourself enough time for travel, exercise, and showering. An hour class could take two hours or more when you factor in the whole experience.

For about a year, Debra attended a Bikram yoga class four to five times a week. This form of yoga was developed by Bikram Choudhury in Los Angeles and is now taught widely in the United States. It consists of 26 poses done in a room heated to about 100 degrees. The class itself was one and a half hours long. Travel each way was about 35 minutes. But to get a spot in the front near the mirror so that she could watch her postural alignment, Debra arrived a half-hour before class started. Yes, her yoga class took over three hours! Fortunately, it was a great class for her and was well worth the time invested. Eventually, her lifestyle changed, with more responsibilities and obligations, and today she couldn't begin to commit that much time so often. She still exercises daily, but now it's at home.

Thinspiration

Every exercise appointment you set is a commitment to yourself. Keep your exercise appointments as sacred as a date with your spouse, attending ball games using your season tickets, or business meetings. Don't make excuses for breaking the dates with yourself. The price is too high. We wish there were an easier way, but there just isn't an alternative to exercising.

Body of Knowledge

The best time of day to exercise is the time that works best for you. There isn't a precise formula for when to exercise. You may find that exercise in the evening keeps you wide awake at bedtime. If so, find another time.

Don't count on "making up" missed exercise appointments. They often never get done for one reason or another. If you're a person who simply doesn't schedule yourself well, perhaps you need to schedule twice as many exercise dates so that you can meet your commitment to yourself. Remember that, with exercise, you aren't accountable to anyone else—only to yourself and your body.

Schedule the time of day that works best for you. If you're not a morning person, planning to be at the gym by 6 A.M. just isn't going to work for long. Perhaps you would enjoy exercising right after work before you go home. Set your appointments for the time of day that works for you. You may also want to break up the time. For example, do 20 minutes or more of aerobics in the morning before you get in the shower; then do your strength training later in the day.

You hardly need to schedule time to do the five Tibetans because they only take 5 minutes (or 10 minutes at most). We figure that doing them should be about as ordinary and routine as brushing your teeth. You just do them.

What to Do

No matter which forms of exercise you choose, here are the minimum amounts you should plan on in a week. By "minimum," we mean the very least you need. However, with exercise—unlike with food—more is often better.

Here is a guideline:

- ◆ Aerobics: 20 minutes daily or 45 minutes three times a week
- ◆ Strength: 30 minutes to an hour twice a week
- ◆ Stretching: 15 to 30 minutes twice a week

Add-Ons

What fun! With exercise, you can vary the routine, learn new ones, and never get bored. Exercise is one area in your life where you can include an almost unlimited number of variations. You're not stuck with just one approach. You can add lots of fun activities to your basic exercise program. These add-ons are, in a sense, "free" treats. There may not be any free foods, but there sure is free exercise. So yes, limit foods but don't limit your exercise. You can fill your "dance card" with fun movement and exercise. In this case, more is better and better for you. Plan on enjoying exercise and recreation so much that you prefer them to just sitting around or rushing around. Your body will thank you.

On the Road

As we said earlier, there are no excuses for not exercising, and that includes business travel and vacations. You don't give up food when you travel, so why would you give up exercise?

Many enlightened hotels and motels have exercise rooms with enough equipment to get your endorphins lifted and your heart rate elevated for 20 minutes or so. If not, well, get creative. Do step-ups on the staircase at equipment-deficient hotels. Yes, it looks weird to the people using the stairs (usually very few folks), but looking weird is better than not exercising.

We know there's a floor in your room, and a floor is all you need to do the five Tibetans. Some hotel rooms have VCRs on which you can play a favorite exercise video. Plus, some exercise videos are now on DVD, which you can view on your laptop.

Some equipment is easy to pack, such as a fitness circle, a fitness ball, or an elastic exercise band. Use these to get in your strength training. We know people who take free weights on the road, but that's beyond the scope of what we're willing to lug through airports.

Thinspiration

Treat exercise on the road as you would eating on the road—make it essential. You'll find that it increases your energy and makes your trip more enjoyable.

Exercise-Altering Conditions

Other things can happen to interrupt your exercise plans. Let's discuss these and find solutions.

Weather

Weather happens. Yucky weather can keep you from walking, jogging, hiking, or swimming. It can even keep you from getting to the gym if the roads are icy. Make sure you have alternative plans. In-home exercising is the obvious solution. Be clever, be smart, and don't let rain, sleet, or snow interfere with your exercise.

Ailments

If you have a seasonal cold or flu, exercise can actually stimulate your immune system and aid your recovery. But be careful not to overdo it. Low-impact activities such as yoga and Pilates are good choices, so you don't need to stay in bed unless the doctor orders it.

Following surgery, take your time to recover. As soon as you can, though, start moving and do as much as you can without injuring yourself. Get your doctor's advice on how soon you can exercise.

> **CAUTION**
>
> **Weighty Warning**
>
> If you're in pretty good shape, your body will recover faster after surgery. But don't rush it. After an emergency appendectomy, Lucy needed two weeks before she could even try the Tibetans. And then it took another two weeks before she could do them all fully. The good news was that her everyday commitment to fitness helped her recover more quickly.

Bodily aches can certainly make exercise unpleasant, and yet the benefits may actually help. Even those suffering from terrible arthritis are encouraged to exercise as much as possible. Check with your doctor and with a sports therapist for what you can do within your current limitations. Often there is plenty.

Sports Injuries

Unfortunately, sports injuries sometimes result from exercise. Should this happen, of course, rest and rehabilitate. You may need to learn new ways of movement so that you can avoid injuries in the future. Most sports rehab involves movement and gradually rebuilding your strength, so you can continue to exercise.

Pregnancy

Yes, you can exercise when pregnant, just carefully. Be sure to check with your doctor before you begin. Then join an exercise class designed for pregnant women or use one of the videos especially for your situation.

Setting Goals

Our favorite adage about goals is to start slow to go fast. Way too often, new exercisers have great expectations about their bodies. Then they pay the price for overdoing it. How about you?

Have you ever gone to an aerobics class at the gym and tried really hard to keep up with the person in front of you? You got an A+ for effort. You gasped for breath and your legs shook from the exertion, but you soldiered on. The next morning and the following day, your body ached unmercifully. Simple activities such as walking and going up stairs seemed next to impossible. Boy, were you asking for it!

Start slowly. Gradually increase your exercise time or intensity to allow your body to adapt. Work up gradually to 20 minutes of cardio/aerobics. Ditto strength training. Ditto stretching.

You can always modify your goals if you want more, and there can be good reasons to want more. You may have a specific objective that you want to focus on. For example, we find that strength training is more helpful to fit into your clothes at 40 or 50 or even 60 years old. Plus the bone-strengthening factor of strength training becomes more significant with age.

Thinspiration

A personal goal helps. Your goal may be to attain an acceptable level of aerobics and maintain it. Your goal may be to climb Mount Everest. Perhaps you want to take up a particular sport or outdoor activity. For most of us, though, just getting in shape, staying in shape, and having fun doing it are plenty.

The Scorecard

Your most important scorecard is how you look and feel, plus how you fit into your clothes. Another important scorecard is how your mood and perspective are lifted as you continue your cardio/aerobics, strengthening, and flexibility program.

We also realize that keeping a tally sheet helps. A rule of thumb in business is that what you count tends to increase. The same is true of exercise. If you count clicks on a pedometer, you'll most likely jog or run more. If you count exercise sessions, you tend to do more of them. With that in mind, we suggest that you keep a weekly and monthly exercise chart.

Weekly Exercise Scorecard

	Cardio/Aerobic		Strength-Training		Flexibility	
	Method	*Duration*	*Method*	*Duration*	*Method*	*Duration*
Monday						
Tuesday						
Wednesday						
Thursday						
Friday						
Saturday						
Sunday						
Total for week						

Thinspiration

When you review your exercise scorecard, if you didn't do as well as you planned, don't become upset with yourself. Forgive yourself and do better the next week, but don't quit keeping score because you'll lessen your resolve.

Put a copy of your scorecard on your desk or in your daily planner. Perhaps tape it to your bathroom mirror. At the end of the week, review how well you did.

Exercise is vital to reaching your ideal size and staying there for life. It gives you energy, soothes stress, and boosts your metabolism. The higher your metabolism, the easier it is to lose weight and keep it off. The less stress you experience, the less stress eating you'll do. Plus, the more energy you have, the easier it is to eat from 0 to 5.

The Least You Need to Know

◆ Decide whether you are better off exercising at home or at a gym based on how each fits with your lifestyle and personality.

◆ Make sure you have an at-home program for the days when you can't get to the gym or when you are on the road.

◆ Keep up your exercise program during vacations and business travel.

◆ Have realistic goals for making progress and continuing the program for life.

◆ Schedule appointments with yourself for exercise and write them in your daily planner.

◆ Keep track of your fitness progress by using a diary, scorecard, or fitness log.

Part 5

Understanding Weight-Loss Plans

Every day, almost everywhere, you're bombarded with advertisements, articles, and hype on the latest diet plan or weight-loss system. Because the U.S. population continues to grow fatter, you can expect to hear about even more weight-loss "solutions."

Few of them offer lasting results. Most offer hope when you're feeling desperate on a chubby Monday morning. Some offer a chance to lose a couple of pounds quickly but little else. Of course, the weight is back the next week.

A couple of approaches to weight loss are real gems. They might just work for you. In this part of the book, we review popular diet plans and show you how to find the jewels amid the hype.

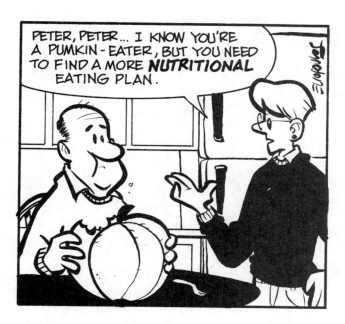

Chapter 19

Choosing a Weight-Loss Plan

In This Chapter

- ◆ Choosing a weight-loss plan you can live with
- ◆ Simple and healthy are best
- ◆ How to sift through the hype
- ◆ Avoiding dangerous diets

Every new weight-loss plan or diet is advertised as "the last one you'll ever need." You know it's just hype, but hope mixed with desperation is a strong motivator. Do you really believe that somehow, with just the right plan—voilà!—you'll miraculously awaken one morning at your ideal size?

Why are we all so silly when it comes to diets? Why do we suspend our common sense and intelligence when we're thinking about losing weight?

There are good weight-loss plans and diets. There are some pretty bad ones, too. A few are even dangerous. Some come with high price tags. Others are virtually free. Still others are outright scams.

In this chapter, we tell you what to look for in a weight-loss plan or diet so that you can make wiser choices. You'll come away with some guidelines to evaluate not just the specific weight-loss approaches we discuss in this book but all future programs for shedding excess fat. We'll use the criteria in the next several chapters as we review popular weight-loss programs.

Monday Madness

I'll start my diet on Monday. We can't really call them "famous last words" because many people who want to lose weight say them over and over again. Monday comes and goes, and the next Monday comes and goes, and soon the dieter is on to yet the next promised miracle. Even when the individual actually does begin dieting on Monday, all bets are off come Friday afternoon. After all, who can diet on the weekend?

When Sandy's co-workers tell her they are going on a diet Monday morning, she laughs and asks them, "And when are you going off it?" She knows, as you do, that Monday morning diets are temporary quick fixes and are born out of frustration and desperation, not from a deeply committed choice to attain a lifestyle of living at one's ideal size.

> **Thinspiration**
>
> The most important factor in a good weight-loss approach is you. Your commitment and perseverance make it work or not. Yes, you need to choose a plan that works with your body and fits into your lifestyle, but no plan is miraculous. You make the difference.

The surest way to reach and stay at your ideal size is to make a conscious and well-thought-out decision to make a significant lifestyle change and stick with it for life. In fact, it may be the only way. Flitting from weight-loss plan to weight-loss plan undermines your efforts and dooms you to perpetual battles of the bulge. Your goal should be to walk away from your weight issue forever, not to revisit the same problem with new approaches every six months.

Think of your weight-loss plan as a means to an end—to reach your ideal size and stay there. Don't experiment with diets and weight-loss plans as if doing so is some kind of hobby. There's nothing special about ringing up a long list of diets that you've *failed* at. Yes, dieting is often part of the office chatter. But wouldn't you rather have folks compliment you for your lifelong success than for losing five pounds quickly on the latest fad diet?

There are some good weight-loss plans that can help you for life, but only if you work the plan. Let's take a look at the critical criteria for choosing good approaches.

Does It Wear Well?

When choosing a weight-loss plan, first consider how it fits into your lifestyle. Few of us want to make dieting the center of our lives. We want eating to be a natural experience that we enjoy the way a naturally thin person enjoys eating. So let's consider some important lifestyle criteria.

Will It Last a Lifetime?

As you examine a weight-loss approach, ask yourself, *"Can I follow this plan day in and day out for the rest of my life?"* It takes lots of emotional energy to start yet another weight-loss eating plan. Make sure the one you choose is worth your effort ... for life! The last thing you want is another failure. Finding a successful lifetime approach to eating will restore your emotional energy and make you feel as if you've mastered a significant aspect of your life—because you have.

Make sure you like the foods you are being asked to eat because you will be eating them for a lifetime. If you don't like cabbage soup, why would you ever choose a diet that features cabbage soup? Eating absolutely should be pleasurable and sensuous. If a weight-loss plan isn't going to delight you, why waste your time? Why waste your emotional energy? Figure that you only have so much emotional energy to spend on a weight-loss plan. If this one's going to be for life, make sure it's worth the effort.

> **Weighty Warning**
>
> You don't want to yo-yo diet for the rest of your life. You've been there, done that. Typically, yo-yo dieting puts you into starvation metabolism, and that always leads to weight gain. Avoid quick weight-loss plans because they bring with them the ensuing quick weight gain.

> **Thinspiration**
>
> Assume that you *will* find a lifelong approach to eating that allows you to reach and stay at your ideal size ... pleasurably. Don't approach your weight-loss plan as a painful chore that you must undertake. Negative thoughts will inevitably lead you to one more dieting failure.

Is It Simple?

How complicated is this weight-loss approach? Generally speaking, the simpler the better. The more complicated the plan, the less likely it is that a person can stay on it indefinitely. You need to be able to live your life while on a weight-loss plan. The more complex your diet and eating plan becomes, the more you will have to sacrifice other aspects of your life. When considering a weight-loss plan, ask the following:

- ◆ Can I eat at regular restaurants?
- ◆ Can I eat at my work desk?
- ◆ Will it be easy to stick to on vacations?
- ◆ Can I eat comfortably at a client lunch?
- ◆ Will I be able to eat at holiday parties?
- ◆ Will my dinner food be the same as my family's?

If you can't enjoy yourself naturally on a plan under these situations, the plan may be too complicated. You should be able to follow it with ease even during the holidays. Yes, this is possible.

Does It Fit How I Live?

Does this weight-loss plan fit into my lifestyle? Your weight-loss plan needs to fit you and how you live.

One man, a golfer, lost 40 pounds on a weight-loss plan centered around a diet shake. To maintain his weight loss, he still drank the shakes for lunch. When he played golf, between the front and back nine, he snuck into the restroom, mixed up his shake, went into one of the stalls, and quickly downed it so that none of his golfing buddies would know. This sure isn't what we had in mind when we said to eat beautifully! Clearly, his weight-loss approach didn't easily fit into his lifestyle; he never shared a burger with the guys in the clubhouse grill. It's sad—and also unnecessary.

> **Thinspiration**
>
> If the weight-loss plan you've chosen embarrasses you when eating in public, it's not the right plan.
> When you choose a plan, determine if you could follow it at a client luncheon, with a prospective boss, or with your best friends.

If you don't like to cook and the weight-loss plan has you tied to the stove, forget it. It won't work for the long haul. If you take weekend camping trips, can you follow the plan out in the wilderness? If you travel on business frequently, can you order the recommended foods at most restaurants and comfortably eat with clients?

Will your family eat the recommended foods so that you don't have to cook two different entrées at every meal? Do you want your children to have to deal with you eating weird foods? Would you be embarrassed eating as the plan recommends at a business luncheon or convention? Can you go out on a date or to dinner with friends and stay faithful to your weight-loss plan?

If you answer "no" to any of these questions, you probably want to find a better approach. In essence, you want a plan that lets you live your life, not one that makes you a slave to unnatural rules and foods.

Work with Your Biology

The weight-loss plan you choose must work with your biology for you to be successful. Some plans do, but an amazing number of weight-loss approaches go against the human body's natural processes for eating, digestion, and nutrition.

Overeating Never Works

First and foremost, make sure the weight-loss plan doesn't advise you to overeat. Yes, there really are approaches that recommend that you gorge yourself on certain foods. However, no food free-for-all can result in healthy weight loss. Avoid any plan that encourages you to violate your stomach space by putting in too much food. If a plan suggests you can eat as much as you want and still lose weight, move on to something else. A person simply can't get thin for life by overeating, no matter whether it's celery, steak, or tomato soup.

Starvation Leads to Weight Gain

Will this weight-loss plan put me into starvation metabolism? This happens if you're not eating enough food in a day to sustain life normally. Starvation diets are often counterproductive and harmful. If you starve yourself, your body responds by going into starvation metabolism, which in turn makes it more difficult to lose weight. (This was covered in more detail in Chapter 6.) Your cravings turn food into the "forbidden fruit" you can't have … an unhealthy attitude that makes you want it even more. This often results in binge eating when you can't take being starved any longer. Starvation diets are typically among the worst yo-yo diets. Any diet labeled "starvation" should likely be avoided.

Starvation diets are unpleasant, hard on the body, and seldom, if ever, effective for lifelong weight maintenance. When your body is deprived of a healthy quantity of food, it shifts into starvation metabolism and begins using your muscles for fuel instead of your stored fat. Starvation diets often lead to headaches, irritability, fatigue, lightheadedness, and other side effects.

Thinspiration

Never abuse your body. Individuals who live comfortably in their bodies never think of food as an enemy. Have confidence that a healthy, balanced diet will support you in reaching your ideal size.

Safety Comes First

How safe is this weight-loss plan? Better health is one of the key reasons you want to lose weight and stay at your ideal size, so it sure doesn't make any sense to endanger your health as you lose weight. Here are some basic safety checks:

◆ Make sure you are advised to eat proteins, fats, and fruits and vegetables daily.

◆ Make sure you aren't advised to take any herbal supplements that are known to be harmful, such as ephedra.

◆ Make sure any prescription medications you're taking are compatible and safe with your chosen plan.

◆ Make sure you aren't supposed to eat foods that you're allergic to.

◆ Make sure the company or weight-loss plan doesn't have pending lawsuits about safety issues.

If anything at all about the weight-loss system seems questionable in terms of safety, be careful. Are you willing to risk the health of your internal organs, a stroke, or even death to lose weight? Since there are safe ways to lose weight, risky approaches are generally not good choices.

Your Health Is Important, Too

Does the weight-loss program promote good health? The really good weight-loss programs focus on health as much as weight loss. Good programs support the lifelong relationship between healthy living and maintaining an ideal body size for life.

However, some plans almost exclusively focus on weight loss … at any cost. For instance, some weight-loss programs rely on high-powered stimulants that can cause anxiety, insomnia, and irritability. Others simply fill you up with nonnutritive bulk fiber. Such plans are *not* designed to sustain your health.

Reaching your ideal size but not living healthfully is just not worth it.

The Price of Weight Loss

How much does the weight-loss plan cost? The cost range is wide. You can find good plans on the Internet at no cost, or you can pay thousands for some clinically supervised plans. Are expensive approaches simply better? Of course not. Plenty of people have lost weight and stayed at their ideal size without tapping into their savings accounts.

Buying a couple of books, going to a seminar, or using nutritional supplements are all reasonable costs. So is investing in exercise videos and equipment or even a health club membership. But it's not essential to purchase expensive supplements or special foods month after month that will ruin your budget.

Thinspiration

Consider other alternatives before you commit a lot of money to a weight-loss plan. You can reach your ideal size without big cash outlays. Wouldn't it be more fun to spend the money on new clothes, vacations, and enjoying your new size?

CAUTION **Weighty Warning** _____

Try not to be guided by your emotions when deciding on a weight-loss program. Some Internet scam artists will try to entice you to send cash for their weight-loss products. They know that frantic dieters make dumb, emotional purchases. Even some well-known, respectable weight-loss plans will play on your emotions. When you're being pitched a weight-loss program, keep your head screwed on and leave your credit card at home. Take at least 24 hours to make your decision.

Many weight-loss programs offer more than just a diet or eating plan. They offer special foods and supplements. There's nothing fundamentally wrong with that, but sometimes it goes too far. Some programs aggressively promote their foods as the best way to lose weight. Others pretty much mandate that you use their foods with their programs.

If you think a ribeye steak is expensive, get ready for sticker shock when you see the price of some weight-loss food! These special foods and supplements are often quite costly. Thus, using them for life becomes a real challenge.

We generally recommend weight-loss systems that work with normal foods that are widely available and avoid those that derive their profits from food sales.

Common Sense Food Suggestions

Weight loss is about eating and food. So when you're looking into weight-loss plans, use your common sense and what you've learned about nutrition to guide your selection process. The good weight-loss programs honor the body and how it works. If a plan's food suggestions don't support healthy nutrition, you won't make progress toward your lifetime goal. You may lose a few pounds temporarily, but that's about all.

Let's discuss some common-sense criteria to apply to weight-loss programs.

Balance Is Important

Will I eat all the essential foods in balance? That is, does the plan recommend about 25 to 35 percent protein, about 30 to 50 percent carbohydrates, and about 20 to 30 percent fats? If not, the plan's meal suggestions are not balanced, and your eating will not be in alignment with

CAUTION **Weighty Warning** _____

A food plan that is unbalanced can lead to starvation metabolism and weight gain. Balanced eating of proteins, fats, and carbohydrates gives you confidence that you can get to your ideal size and stay there for life.

your body's basic nutritional needs. Unbalanced eating is unhealthy as a lifetime approach. We even question whether a couple weeks of unbalanced eating serves your weight-loss goals because it can put you into starvation metabolism. Beware any weight-loss program that ignores the basics of good nutrition. You will likely pay for it later.

The Fresh Five

Will I get to eat fruits and vegetables? Make sure the weight-loss program encourages you to eat lots of fresh fruits and vegetables, preferably a minimum of five servings every day. Fruits and vegetables are so fundamentally good for you that any plan that doesn't encourage eating them is immediately suspect. Any plan that actually discourages you from eating fruits and vegetables is unhealthy.

Also, make sure you're encouraged to have variety in those servings. Five servings of bananas or five servings of cabbage per day are not even close to the essence of the recommendation. Ditto for watermelon.

Eat Versus Drink

Are liquid diets good or bad for me? There's a lot to be said for actually eating. It's quite natural and satisfying. Putting food in our mouths, chewing, and swallowing feel good. Plus, the saliva used during chewing is the starting point for good digestion. It's also easier to feel your hunger numbers when you sit down and chew your food slowly. Drinking skips over some of these steps, and research shows that your overall caloric intake may go up because your body is less satisfied from drinking compared to eating. Plus, there's a good chance you're drinking a concoction that's loaded with highly refined ingredients that are high glycemic, something we always discourage. For a refresher on high- versus low-glycemic eating, refer to Chapter 9. We favor weight-loss programs that encourage you to eat and chew. Drinking your food once in a while, as in a shake, is fine, but please don't do it every day and especially never more than once a day. And never do it if you don't like the taste!

Body of Knowledge

The word is finally out that some fat is good for you. Be sure that any weight-loss system you use allows at least 15 percent fat and up to 30 percent in your overall diet. If it recommends essential fatty acids, all the better.

Get Enough Fat

The weight-loss system you choose should recommend enough fat to keep you healthy and to let your body release fat stores. Eating less than 15 percent fat is not good. The better plans also urge you to get plenty of essential fatty acids every day.

If the plan is fat-aphobic, find another one.

Avoid Processed Starches

Truthfully, we've never found a plan that actually forces you to eat bagels and white bread, and none of them tout cookies and cakes as your path to weight-loss nirvana. However, some of them recommend that you frequently eat processed low-fat foods that contain high-glycemic carbohydrates. Avoid these plans.

Accessible Foods

Can I purchase the recommended foods at the grocery store or a nearby health food store? Are the foods easy to find, easy to cook, and easy to pay for? If your plan recommends fresh frog legs, well, we suspect it will be hard to sustain for most of us. Exotic foods are wonderful in many ways and certainly you can enjoy them, but they aren't necessary for successful weight loss. It's too much work and too hard to sustain over time.

Maintenance Is Key

Will I be able to maintain this plan for life? Your weight-loss efforts are wasted if you can't easily maintain your new ideal size. With any weight-loss program, check out the maintenance plan included. These typically come in a few varieties:

The maintenance plan encourages you to keep doing what you're doing. In other words, the basic plan and the maintenance plan are the same thing. This is absolutely the best kind of maintenance plan because you can use the program for life. But it needs to be balanced and simple.

The maintenance program gradually adds in more foods and variety. If you start to gain weight, you revert back to the original program. We see less success with this approach. If the original program had lots of restrictions, it may have put you into both physical and emotional starvation mode. When you can finally return to regular eating, your tendency is to eat excessively and make up for lost time and missed food.

No maintenance plan is offered. The program just ends with no continuing help. You can probably count on regaining your weight.

What If You Don't Want to Eat at All?

Some of you may have decided you just don't want to deal with food. Or meals. Or eating. At all. Of course, avoiding food isn't a viable long-term solution to your weight problem. You may feel you are out of control with food, so you want to quit cold turkey. People who have addictions, such as alcoholics and substance abusers, can

Thinspiration

You don't need to stay constantly afraid of gaining weight when you eat. By eating 0 to 5 and consuming balanced and nutritious meals, you will make peace with food and eating and lose your fear of food. Remember, food doesn't make you fat; overeating food makes you fat. You can and will succeed!

totally avoid those substances for life. You can't avoid food. You need it to survive.

Yes, you're tired of battling your weight issue, but it really is possible to develop a personal, healthy approach to eating. If you use the criteria identified in this chapter, you'll be able to find an approach that leaves you energized, happy, and at your ideal size. But please choose a weight-control system cautiously, just as you would choose a home, a relationship, or a career. Reaching and staying at your ideal size for life is a life-changing experience. We want you to have the best. Be selective. Be picky.

The Least You Need to Know

- ◆ Select a weight-loss program with a watchful eye toward health, safety, and practicality.

- ◆ Seek out a program that will work for you, your lifestyle, and the long term.

- ◆ Avoid any plans that put you into starvation metabolism or that go against your natural biology.

- ◆ Carefully consider the overall lifetime cost before making a commitment.

- ◆ Be picky about choosing a weight-loss program because you deserve only the best.

Chapter 20

Rating Diet Systems

In This Chapter

- Evaluating the classic weight-loss programs
- Criteria for selecting any program
- The problems with prepackaged diet foods
- Getting the most from the Internet

Diets of one kind or another are still going strong. While our Paleolithic ancestors probably didn't fret over extra pounds, that's certainly not true in modern times. Diets have been around throughout the twentieth century and now into the twenty-first century. You can be pretty sure they'll still be around in the next century, too.

Since at least the 1950s, Americans have turned to others for help in shedding pounds and keeping them off. We've wanted someone to give us a "plan" that will do the trick. Hence, today there are a bunch of organized weight-loss programs. And yes, they've guided many people to their ideal size, at least for a while and some for life.

There's much good to be said for weight-loss programs. Most of the time, they're sensible and focus on your lifelong quest to reach and stay at your ideal size. Typically, their meal plans are pretty balanced, with an emphasis on the eating guidelines of the classic food pyramid. Today, several of these plans have updated themselves and introduced terrific websites that support their users.

Unfortunately, just because some weight-loss programs have been around for decades, it doesn't mean they're right for you. We think some of them have real problems. Let's take a closer look.

Buy Our Food, Lose Weight ... Right?

Some of the best-known *diet systems* offer prepackaged foods. Why? Because you need help. Right? Out of desperation, you don't even want to think about what and how to eat. "Just tell me what to do!" you cry out.

Prepackaged foods are touted as the ideal conven-ience. They offer portion control and the "right" kinds of food. On the surface, it makes perfectly good sense that you would turn to someone to tell you what to eat because you haven't succeeded on you own. Plus, these systems also offer various kinds of psychological support to make your new eating regimen more palatable.

Let's look at how well these systems might or might not work for you in attaining and maintaining your ideal size for life while eating for health and energy.

Lean Lingo

A weight-loss program, sometimes known as a **diet sys-tem,** is primarily an organized eating plan to assist you in losing weight and keeping it off. Typically they offer very specific suggestions for what foods to eat, how often to eat, portion control, and other eating "rules." Some of the best-known plans offer their own prepackaged foods or special supplements.

Weighty Warning

You can get to your ideal size and stay there for life by eating regular foods. Special diet foods are not the answer to anyone's weight-loss problems. Be sure that any plan you choose stands on its own without "diet" foods or shakes.

Weight Watchers

Weight Watchers is practically a household name. The company has been in business for about 40 years and is most famous for its weekly weigh-in meetings. At these meetings, members weigh themselves in a group setting, receiving "hurrahs!" from other mem-bers when they show progress and lots of emotional support when they don't.

As Weight Watchers has grown, it has added a monthly magazine, processed foods and meals that are available in grocery stores, and a website that's useful and informative.

Weight Watchers brand prepackaged food may offer portion control, but it's far from ideal. It overemphasizes low fat and is high glycemic. Plus, it's loaded with heavily processed foods and preservatives. Not good. We don't recommend that you eat Weight Watchers food products. Fortunately, you don't have to. You can still take advantage of the weekly support groups.

Weight Watchers has dramatically revised its recommended eating plan. There was a time when each member weighed and measured all food and could only eat so much of certain types of food at every meal. It was a very regimented eating system.

Today, Weight Watchers uses a point system. Based on a person's desired weight and other factors, each member is given a certain number of points to eat each day. This way, a person can have a piece of cake or ice cream and still lose weight. So far, so good. You can choose the best ratios of protein, fats, and carbs for you. We also like this.

Weight Watchers designates some foods as "free foods," meaning you can eat them whenever you want with no limit to quantity. Typically, free foods are raw vegetables such as celery, cabbage, and radishes. We discourage you from overeating any food, even vegetables.

One of our concerns with the Weight Watchers point system is that you can get too hungry! Nancy was a member of Weight Watchers who thought she would like the simple "organization" of a point system. But most days she ate all her points for the day by noon. From noon on, she wouldn't eat again until the next morning. At dinner, she would sit with her family while they ate the dinner she cooked. Sure, she could eat a plate full of celery while they ate a robust meal, but that seemed less appealing than not eating at all … especially after the fourth or fifth dinner! One day Nancy realized that the unconscious messages she was sending to her family, especially her teenaged daughter, were not healthy.

Many serious eating disorders, such as bulimia and anorexia, are rooted in a parent's conscious and unconscious messages to the child about weight and eating. Nancy was silently telling her daughter that it was okay to put her body into extreme hunger for the sake of sticking to her diet (and that it was okay to follow rigid eating rituals). Nancy didn't want her daughter to emulate her eating and develop both weight and eating issues, so she quit the program.

> **Thinspiration**
>
> Food isn't the enemy. Any diet system that causes you to "starve" yourself during even part of the day creates an unhealthy attitude about eating. Food itself becomes evil, and all foods become "forbidden fruit." Often this leads to starvation metabolism and subsequent binge eating.

Weight Watchers seems to move a bit slowly in response to current nutritional research. It still recommends that you eat processed foods and highly refined carbohydrates. It subscribes to a low-fat, high-glycemic eating approach and does not encourage members to get plenty of essential fatty acids every day.

That said, the support system is very helpful. You can even "go to meetings" online, which means you can save your evenings for family and fun. We like this.

Weight Watchers strongly encourages exercise and does a great job of showing members how to put together home programs.

Its maintenance program is challenging to stick with, as is any maintenance plan that differs from the diet plan. As with all dieters who rebound from restricted calorie intake, a member's tendency is to go overboard and make up for lost time. Easing into normal eating is quite challenging and not as successful as the original weight-loss results.

If you choose to use Weight Watchers, we encourage you to always eat 0 to 5 and not consider any food to be a free food. Avoid the company's prepackaged meals and foods. Take your essential fatty acids every day and avoid high-glycemic starches. Eat at least 40 grams of high-quality protein every day. Get the most out of Weight Watchers's support and exercise suggestions.

Jenny Craig

The cost of the Jenny Craig system gets in the way of anything good it offers. To use the Jenny Craig System, you're supposed to eat its prepackaged foods. As you might guess, these foods are highly processed with low-fat and high-glycemic carbs and contain artificial ingredients such as preservatives. At a cost of about $90 a week, your tab will come to about $400 for the month. Plus you still have to buy fresh fruits and vegetables, some side foods, and also feed your family. Ouch!

> **Body of Knowledge**
>
> Some formal weight-loss plans are great for delivering motivation and support. They can help you stay on course and avoid discouragement, but sometimes the regimentation interferes with your healthy and common sense approach to food and eating.

Needless to say, most of us can't eat this way over a lifetime ... even if we put a second mortgage on the house to pay for it! However, several of our friends have maintained a lifetime relationship with Jenny Craig. They return every couple of years to lose the 75-plus pounds they've packed on since their last go around with Jenny Craig.

For all its cost, Jenny Craig foods can be very skimpy. The average breakfast entrée only offers 3 to 4 grams of protein. Hardly enough. We recommend about 15 grams. Weekly weigh-ins and counseling are part of the program. The cost for joining varies, but it's minimal compared to the cost of the food.

Eating Jenny Craig foods creates a dependence on the products that makes it difficult to return to eating regular foods.

Most customers join out of a desperate desire to have a systematic approach they can use to shed pounds quickly. We don't recommend the Jenny Craig program.

Evaluating Other Weight-Loss Programs

Just look in your local phone book to find many more weight-loss centers and programs. Before you visit them, call and ask the following questions to determine if you should even consider visiting. The sales reps will often urge you to come in and talk because they know how to sell you when you are there in person. It's hard to ask analytical questions once the box of Kleenex comes out and you're in the throes of emotion. So resist the sales rep's urging and try to get answers to these questions before you visit:

Question	Preferred Answer
Do you offer prepackaged foods, and do I need to eat them?	No, we want you to eat your own food.
Do I have to weigh?	No.
Does the plan encourage or discourage me from skipping meals or not eating for periods of time?	We discourage any kind of starvation mode. We make sure you get adequate food on a day-to-day basis to keep your metabolism and energy high.
Do you recommend low-glycemic eating?	Yes, we do.
Do I have to eat low fat?	No, we recognize the importance of healthy dietary fats and recommend that you keep fat intake between 15 and 30 percent.
Do you recommend that I take essential fatty acids?	Yes, EFAs will help you burn excess fat.
Do you recommend I use a hunger scale?	Yes, we want you to learn how to know your body and honor its hunger needs.
Is there a maintenance plan?	The plan you'll use to get to your ideal size is basically the same one you'll use to stay there.

continues

continued

Question	Preferred Answer
Do you suggest I use any products containing ephedra, ma huang, or country mallow? (More information on these products in Chapter 24.)	No, for health reasons, we don't promote their use.
Do you suggest I use bulking agents so that I feel full?	No, we don't use them.
Does your program include soy shakes or protein drinks?	No, our program doesn't. You can use them occasionally if you want.
Do you recommend an exercise program?	Yes, we'll help you design one that suits you and your lifestyle.
How fast can I lose my weight?	We don't encourage fast weight loss but rather genuine, slow loss that stays off. We know the dangers of yo-yo dieting and want you to avoid it.
Do you recommend that I use artificial sweeteners such as aspartame, saccharine, or Splenda?	Generally not. They are okay in small amounts, say one or two servings a week and only when necessary for a person who for medical reasons can't have sugar—such as a diabetic.
Can you give me the names of several people who have used your system? I would like to call them. I want to talk with a couple of people who were successful and some who were not.	We don't give out client names, but we can ask several to phone you.

Only after a weight-loss program answers these questions to your satisfaction should you consider setting up a meeting. When you do go, stay alert. Consider other alternatives and don't sign anything on your first visit.

Weighty Warning _____

Before you visit a weight-loss program or diet center, pause and ask yourself why you are going. Is it for motivational support? If so, maybe the program will help. Or is it because you can't control your own eating and need to be forced into a rigid plan? If so, the weight-loss system may not be adequate to help you stay at your ideal size for life. You may be setting yourself up for one more yo-yo dieting failure.

Overeaters Anonymous

Overeaters Anonymous is a not-for-profit organization that offers support groups to assist people who are overweight and obese. Their premise is that overeating is an addiction and a disease. The program uses a 12-step approach adapted from Alcoholics Anonymous.

The meetings are free with donations welcome. You can attend as many as you want. Overeaters Anonymous encourages members to avoid sugars and other designated "addictive" foods. They support balanced meals and wholesome nutrition.

We question whether the addiction and disease model works well for overeating. An alcoholic can abstain forever from drinking; however, a person can't abstain from eating. At each meeting, visitors introduce themselves by saying, "My name is (*state first name only*), and I am a compulsive overeater."

Therein lies our biggest problem with Overeaters Anonymous. We don't believe that once a person is a compulsive overeater, he or she is forever a compulsive overeater.

While overeating often involves powerful underlying psychological issues, we don't believe overeating should be classified with alcoholism. Saying this statement aloud is a very strong affirmation. Studies show that what a person thinks and says is often a self-fulfilling prophecy. Certainly, the spiritual focus at the group meetings is valuable, and the group support can be terrific. But overall, we suggest you use a more positively focused program.

Thinspiration

Please don't ever call yourself a "compulsive overeater." Instead, affirm your positive self-image. Say, "I am now at my ideal size. I easily master my weight and my eating." You'll learn more about affirmations in Part 6.

Web-Based Eating Plans

The web and weight loss are quickly becoming linked. It's really quite exciting how you can now use the Internet to assist you with weight loss. Even though the web as a tool for weight loss is relatively new, it offers some powerful new approaches. For instance, by first surveying your vital statistics and food preferences, you can get a customized eating plan. Plus, you can get support and information online. Some of the weight-loss sites are great. But watch out, some are really bad.

Watch Out for E-Miracles

By now, you and everyone else with a web connection have received unsolicited e-mails promoting the latest diet craze. Talk about the weight-loss promised land! Whew! You're offered "guaranteed" miracles to shed pounds effortlessly. All you need to do is send cash. Yes, some say, only send cash. Oh, come on. If any of these e-mail solicitations had discovered a miracle approach for weight loss, you'd be reading about it in the newspapers and seeing it on *60 Minutes*. Please don't send them money. The promoters know your vulnerability.

The Really Good Web-Based Programs

Now for the good web-based weight-loss programs. As of the time of this writing, there were several. You may discover others in your web searching. We like these:

- eDiets
- CyberDiets
- iVillage

Weighty Warning

Web-based weight-loss sites may make recommendations for eating based on formulas that aren't right for you. For instance, the formula may recommend a caloric intake that leaves you undernourished, perhaps sending you into starvation metabolism. Apply caution and common sense when using automated weight-loss plans.

Body of Knowledge

You can find registered dietitians who counsel on the web by doing a search for the keyword "dietitian." You can also go to the American Dietetic Association site at www.eatright.org to find a dietitian located near you.

They generally offer a balanced and sensible approach. Many are free, and if not, the cost is minimal. They offer chat rooms for support and exercise recommendations. Some even chart your progress for you. They may offer recommended eating plans and caloric intake, but because the plans are driven by formulas built into their programming, you'll need to determine whether the plan really makes sense for you. The good sites use registered dietitians for counseling and information. They send frequent e-mail newsletters for news and encouragement.

We like many of the sites because they help you deal with stress and emotional eating. Just think, when you want to eat when you aren't hungry, you can just go online and get instant support! You don't need to wait for a friend to return your calls—just get online.

As you check out weight-loss websites, look for the ones that feel good to you. Use the info that makes sense to you and toss the rest. Remember, only you know what works for your body.

The Least You Need to Know

- ◆ If you want to use a diet system, make sure it meets your standards.

- ◆ Avoid eating prepackaged diet foods; they're typically high glycemic and highly processed.

- ◆ Emotional support and encouragement, plus exercise coaching, are often the better features of weight-loss programs.

- ◆ Take advantage of Internet sites for weight-loss support.

- ◆ Just delete those unsolicited e-mails for the newest miracle weight-loss products.

Chapter 21

Food and Eating Philosophies

In This Chapter

◆ Fasting to lose weight

◆ Vegetarianism and weight loss

◆ Other philosophical eating approaches

◆ Eating concepts that better fit your biological needs

Throughout the ages, food has served cultural purposes that go beyond sustenance and pleasure. In many religions, rituals and rules cover many aspects of eating. Some religions restrict certain kinds of foods; some govern how food is prepared and when it can be eaten.

In some religions, food—or fasting from food—is used for ritual purification or as a way to seek higher levels of holiness. For many ages, food has been considered a source for healing and for boosting energy and longevity.

Philosophical approaches to eating add an extra layer—and sometimes extra pounds—to the challenge of reaching your ideal size. Today, many people use these methods for weight loss, although, in general, their origins had nothing to do with weight management. Remember, just because a food ritual has been used for religious reasons for hundreds of years doesn't automatically make it better nutritionally. In this chapter, we will explore both ancient and modern food philosophies.

Fasting

If your religion mandates that you fast as a spiritual practice, by all means, follow the precepts of your chosen religion. *Fasting* for spiritual reasons is a traditional part of the Catholic, Jewish, Hindu, and Muslim faiths, as well as many others. Most of these incorporate fasting as part of special rituals or religious holidays.

If you fast, we hope it is because you are following a traditional religion and not the modern day "religion" of dieting and weight loss. But if you're fasting as a way to lose weight or to control your weight, you may have noticed it doesn't seem to be working. Let's talk about why.

Fasting is usually done by avoiding solid or nutritive foods and most liquids. Water, or perhaps juice, is all that's allowed. By not eating when your body is hungry and by not eating balanced meals, even for a day, you put your body into starvation metabolism. In starvation metabolism, your body slows down metabolically and starts hoarding fat so that you don't starve to death. As you learned earlier in the book, your biological programming for starvation metabolism is strong and resolute. Remember that the body doesn't know how long the fast is going to last, so it prepares for the worst. You know that the fast will last only a day or a couple of days, but your body doesn't.

Fasting is an especially tricky problem for the many overweight people who have low blood sugar. Going without food for longer than four to five hours makes them weak, nauseous, and irritable rather than energized and happy. For these folks, when the fast is finally over, they often binge eat to feel better.

One well-meaning woman, Sylvia, like may others, believed that fasting was a good way to let her digestion rest, to detoxify her body, and to drop a couple of pounds. Her fasting was not based on the precepts of any religion to which she belonged. All she would allow herself was water and two glasses of orange juice for three days. To detoxify, however, the liver needs high-quality protein, the digestive system

> **Lean Lingo**
>
> **Fasting** is the act of abstaining from eating for a period of time, usually one or more days. Often a person ingests only water or juice during this time.

> **Weighty Warning**
>
> Beware using fasting as a weight-loss method. It isn't healthy and can cause more problems than you want to deal with, such as binge eating and weight gain.

doesn't really need rest, and most of the pounds she lost were regained within a day or two after she resumed eating. Fruit juice just isn't the same thing as high-quality protein and essential fatty acids.

Sylvia was one of the many people who fast as a way to lose weight. They fast every month or so. Because fasters sometimes step on the scale at the end of the fast and see that a few pounds have been lost, they keep coming back. Not smart. Fasting to lose weight brings on unnecessary problems—starvation metabolism, weakness, binge eating, and a return of the lost pounds. There are better ways to get to your ideal size.

We don't recommend fasting. In fact, we urge you to avoid fasting for weight loss. It isn't healthy.

Vegetarianism

Vegetarianism began as a religious practice many thousands of years ago. Here's how it all began. In hot climates, such as India, people who ate meat from hoofed animals, meaning cattle and pigs, often became painfully sick and died. When people ate fish and poultry, this didn't happen. Why? Because fish and chicken could be killed and prepared to feed a family for a particular meal. But a whole slaughtered cow or pig couldn't be eaten in one day. Since there was no refrigeration, the leftover meat putrefied quickly. The leftovers were poisonous, to say the least.

In colder climates, such as northern Europe and Asia and the Americas, meat could be safely eaten for several days because it was cold outside much of the year. Also, the indigenous people dried meat and fish—as in beef jerky—to eat later. In hot climates, the meat would have putrefied before it could be dried.

In India, as a way to keep people from eating the beef and pork, the priests and elders declared the cow to be sacred and the pig unclean. Over the years, these eating restrictions became incorporated into today's Hindu religion. Similar food restrictions became part of other religions in hot climates where the cow and pig were indigenous.

Modern-Day Vegetarianism

Vegetarianism today isn't the same. As you can see, religious vegetarianism was rooted in a practical, common sense solution to a deadly situation. With today's refrigeration, these eating rules could be loosened, but since they are tied to established religious doctrine, that won't likely occur.

Vegetarianism today has almost become its own religion, with many varied "sects." Over the past several decades, many people have avoided meat as a path to holiness or higher spiritual experiences. Others avoid eating meat for personal ethical reasons, refusing to support the slaughter of four-legged animals for food. Others avoid meat because they believe it is unnatural or unhealthy to eat. For some, vegetarianism becomes wrapped up in their political views of the world. Unfortunately, many think it's a great way to lose weight. It's not.

There are five broad categories of vegetarians, with lots of personal variations:

- **Vegans** avoid all animal products (meaning meat, fish, poultry, eggs, milk, cheese, and other dairy products), even the wearing of leather shoes.

- **Nonmeat vegetarians** eat eggs, dairy, and fish but not the meat from four-legged animals.

- **Lacto-vegetarians** avoid meat, poultry, fish, and eggs but eat dairy products.

- **Ovo-lacto vegetarians** eat eggs and dairy products but not poultry, fish, or meat from other animals.

- **Semi-vegetarians** mostly follow a vegetarian plan with occasional intakes of meat, poultry, or fish.

Sometimes a person's choice is based on religious rules, sometimes on perceived health benefits, and sometimes on judgments about the ethical issues involved with killing certain kinds of animals for food.

Vegetarianism and Weight Loss

Strict vegetarianism as a lifestyle practice is fine, but don't expect it to be an enlightened path to weight loss. We see too many vegetarian clients with stubborn weight-loss problems to recommend it for losing weight. However, vegetarians who eat at least fish and fowl can get to their ideal size by eating the balanced food plan recommended in Part 3.

If a person's vegetarian preferences are more extreme, it can be nearly impossible to lose weight and keep it off. Eating eggs and cheese can get truly boring, and you have to eat lots of them to get enough complete high-quality protein—like a couple dozen eggs a week and several pounds of cheese! We question the wisdom of this because of the lack of variety, plus constantly eating the same foods invites allergies.

Vegans have an even tougher time losing weight. Vegans regularly fail to get enough complete high-quality protein, and they tend to eat lots of starches, which can really pack on the weight.

Sally was a member of the Hari Krishna religious group for over seven years. With Hindu roots, the sect promotes strict vegetarianism. When I asked how she handled eating no meat for all those years, she replied, "I am a vegetarian in spirit and philosophy, but my body isn't. So I eat meat because my body needs it."

Many of our clients have found that when they add animal protein back into their diets, the weight comes off and they can maintain their ideal size. If you are vegetarian and you can't lose weight, we strongly urge you to start introducing fish, poultry, and meat into your diet until you are eating about 15 to 20 grams of animal protein three times a day.

Weighty Warning

Strict vegetarians often struggle with other health issues besides stubborn body fat. Often their hair, nails, night vision, and skin are less than healthy. Many complain of low energy, which often results in binge eating to compensate. Sometimes supplements can offset the lost nutrients and micronutrients, but basically their bodies are craving high-quality protein.

While we respect philosophical vegetarianism, we also believe that eating meat respects our human nature. Eating animal protein can also be an ethical, philosophical approach to food.

Thinspiration

In one of her many attempts to lose weight, Lucy adopted a totally vegetarian macrobiotic diet. She worked with a macrobiotic specialist who guided her food choices. After 4 months she had gained another 20 pounds, and her husband, who was already quite thin, lost about 20 pounds. Her four-year-old son, Brian, complained of being too tired to walk around the block. Lucy rushed him to the pediatrician.

The diagnosis was anemia. When she told the pediatrician about the family's commitment to macrobiotic eating, he became enraged. Right there, in the waiting room, he loudly commanded her to stop at the grocery store on the way home, buy steaks and a cast iron skillet, and "feed her family and not ever let that child become anemic again."

Within a month, Lucy's 20 pounds were gone, her husband got his weight back up, and her son was his normal—highly active—self. When Brain turned 16, he advised his mom that he was going to become a vegetarian. Her response was, "Over my dead body and yours." Then she told him about his earlier run-in with vegetarian-induced anemia. He changed his mind.

Lucy's weight loss of 20 pounds in a month wasn't the result of going on a diet. Instead, the weight simply fell off when she got out of starvation metabolism.

The Blood-Type Philosophy

Can eating foods in harmony with your blood type assist you in losing weight? That's the premise of the blood-type diet. Proponents also claim that a person can eliminate allergies and improve health.

These theories haven't been substantiated by scientific evidence or through research studies. On the whole, the blood-type diet recommends eating healthy foods and avoiding artificial foods and highly processed and refined carbohydrates. But some of the food recommendations are challenging, to say the least.

Many of our clients have tried the program with limited success. A few find that it works for them really well, but this is a very small percentage.

When you're on the blood-type diet, it's difficult to live a normal life, eat with your family, vacation, go on business trips, and eat in restaurants. When you consider some of the unusual foods that are recommended, you can easily see why. Depending on your blood type, you might be encouraged to eat such foods as rabbit, Ezekiel bread, and quinoa flour.

We don't have a problem with the overall concept or the eating recommendations themselves. We just can't imagine how a person could follow this program for a lifetime.

> **Body of Knowledge**
>
> The blood-type diet recommends that people with type B blood eat lots of rabbit but not eat chicken. Try finding rabbit at a fast-food restaurant! Even lamb, recommended for those with type B and AB blood, is darned hard to find when traveling or eating out with friends.

Food Combining Craziness

Food combining is an unusual concept for weight loss, although variations of this diet have been around since the 1930s. The premise is that certain foods don't digest well when you eat them with certain other foods. When you eat just the right foods in the right combinations, your weight will fall off.

In a nutshell, proteins shouldn't be eaten with starches, and fruits shouldn't be eaten with either proteins or starches. So a person could have meat and vegetables, or veggies and starches, or fruit all by itself. Not surprisingly, there's no scientific evidence to back up these digestion claims.

This diet system is sort of crazy. For instance, it recommends that you eat only fruits for the first 10 days and plenty of them. Obviously, this encourages you to overeat (that is, to eat beyond a 5 on the hunger scale). On day 11, you're told to eat a half-pound of bread, two tablespoons of butter, and three ears of corn. On day 19, you can have some complete protein. Obviously, the plan is unbalanced and will likely result in you missing essential nutrients, essential amino acids, and essential fatty acids.

This diet is a gimmick, is not in alignment with balanced nutrition, and can be dangerous to your health. It will cause your insulin levels to swing wildly and can put you into starvation metabolism, which causes fat storage and, ultimately, regaining any weight you've lost.

Thinspiration

The craziness of the food-combining diet should immediately raise a red flag that warns you to look elsewhere. Use your common sense when evaluating eating systems. Ask yourself, "Is this how my naturally thin friends eat?" Most people who are at their ideal size eat balanced, nutritious diets.

Please, forget food combining. You can do better for your health and still attain your ideal size.

Eat as Paleo Man

To eat as the cavemen did is a simple concept: Your diet should focus on the foods that our Paleolithic ancestors ate. Why? Because our bodies are basically the same as our primitive ancestors' bodies, so our diets should mirror theirs. The DNA of humans has changed less than 0.02 percent over the past 40,000 years. By contrast, grains (such as wheat and corn) were introduced into humankind's diet only about 10,000 years ago. In many parts of the world, some grains and other starches have only been added to the local diets in the past few thousand years.

In our opinion, by adopting the food intake of your ancient ancestors, you could improve your health and get to your ideal size.

One of the best-known primitive eating programs recommends that you eat lean meats, seafood, fish and eggs, plus plenty of fresh fruits and nonstarchy vegetables. You eliminate all dairy, grains, legumes, sugar, and processed and artificial foods. The proportions of proteins, fats, and fruits and vegetables are close to what we recommend in Part 3.

You can eat as a caveman almost anywhere—at restaurants, at cocktail parties, and at a business lunch—although we suggest you use a few modern tools when you do, like a fork and knife instead of your fingers! The maintenance program is the same as the initial eating program, so the plan can work for your lifetime.

One important caution here: The plan is strict. Too strict, in our opinion. It leaves little room for a piece of pizza, a chocolate bar, or a scoop of ice cream. However, we

CAUTION

Weighty Warning

If a primitive eating program advocates eating as much as you want of permitted foods, don't take the advice. You should always tune into your stomach's hunger signals to know when to eat and when to stop eating.

feel that if you could eat the Paleo diet 80 percent of the time, you would be doing your size and health a favor.

You can use the basic insights of the Paleo Diet without becoming philosophically obsessed with it. Use common sense and don't make your treat foods into something bad or evil. Just eat them in moderation, as you would anything else. If the caveman had discovered chocolate 40,000 years ago, you can be sure he would have eaten some!

The Frequent-Eater Plans

These plans claim that the secret to weight loss lies in eating frequently. Most recommend about six small meals a day, usually a healthy mix of proteins, fats, and fruits and vegetables at every meal.

We like the balanced diet, but if you choose a frequent-eater plan, make sure you only eat when you are hungry and stop when you are satisfied (that is, eat when you're at 0 and stop at or below a 5). If it is time for one of your small meals and you are not hungry, wait until you are. There is no benefit in eating when you aren't hungry.

Some of the frequent-eater plans suggest you graze, which means you eat little bits of food all day long. Eating constantly works well for mammals such as cows and sheep, but it doesn't work the same way for humans. Your biology is not that of a ruminating animal. If it were, you also would have four stomachs and a cud. Just think of the exercise effort you would expend trying to keep all four tummies flat!

The Least You Need to Know

- ◆ Fasting for weight loss is usually ineffective and unhealthy.
- ◆ The more strict a vegetarian diet is, the more difficult it becomes to lose weight.
- ◆ Any food plan that is unbalanced or too difficult to maintain isn't going to work over the long term.
- ◆ If your food philosophy is making you fat or unhealthy, stop using it and make a change.

22

Review of Diet Ideas

In This Chapter

- High protein vs. low fat
- Do weight-burning foods exist?
- Eating in the "zone"
- Judging specialty diets

With so many diets out there, how could you possibly choose? One says to avoid fat. The next one says to eat tons of lean protein. Another will tell you to eat lots of protein and fats but no carbohydrates. Yet another will tell you to eat in a "zone." How can all of these approaches possibly work?

The answer is simple. On any given day, for some people, each of these diets work. We'll even bet that a few of them have worked for you … for awhile. We're betting you're ready to get off the diet treadmill. Rather than having to choose your next diet and then the one after that, you want to settle at your ideal size and stay there for life. Let's see how some of these diet approaches stack up for long-term weight loss and health.

High-Protein Diets

Virtually everyone has tried some kind of high-protein diet. The most extreme plans encourage you to eat lots of meat, seafood, and fat and to

Weighty Warnings

The promise of quick weight loss from eating high protein/low carb masks the serious health dangers posed if taken to an extreme. You lose muscle mass, go into potentially harmful ketosis, and usually regain your weight—and more—really fast.

avoid carbohydrates, even fruits and vegetables. In fact, the advocates of these eating plans want you to scrape the breading off your fish in a restaurant. You can eat as much meat and fat as you want provided you eat virtually no carbohydrates. Of course, you won't get fiber in your diet either.

Avoiding all carbohydrates forces the body to find other sources of fuel, so the body will burn body fat for energy. So far, so good. But your body will also break down muscle protein to make glucose for energy. This is called glucogenesis. Your body uses muscle protein from all body muscles—the thighs, the arms, even the heart.

When your body burns fat while deprived of dietary carbohydrates, your body produces ketones. This activity is called *ketosis*. Ketosis does cause weight loss—mostly water weight. The high-protein diets that cause ketosis can be damaging to a person who already has liver or kidney damage.

High-protein diets often cause a big drop in insulin levels, making a person increasingly hungry. With all this going on with high-protein, low-carbohydrate diets, is it any wonder that people tend to regain their weight quickly when the diet is over?

When the diet is over, they have less muscle mass, their brains have struggled to get enough glucose throughout the diet, and they were in the potentially health-threatening state of ketosis. Plus, the loss in muscle mass equates to flabbier muscles. A person can't sustain this way of eating over a lifetime.

Lean Lingo

Ketosis is a body state that occurs when you burn fat without enough glucose. This happens when your diet is low in carbohydrates. Ketosis puts the body under stress and can lead to serious medical complications.

Is it worth it? Absolutely not. The high-protein diet taken to the extreme without any carbs is unhealthy. It lacks nutrient balance, fruits and vegetables, healthy fats, fiber, and we think common sense. The high-protein diets recommend overeating, which always creates problems.

Weight-Burning Foods

Ahhh, those "magic" foods. If only weight loss were so simple. No single food will ever make your body burn enough fat to get you to your ideal size for life. Most will have no positive impact at all. So forget about relying on grapefruit, watermelon, or celery. The same with cabbage soup or any other specific food. All of these may be yummy foods to you, and they're terrific as part of a balanced eating plan, but they hold no magic.

Simple common sense should tell you that reliance on a particular food to get to your ideal size is doomed from the beginning. If you aren't eating a balanced diet, you aren't going to feel energized and healthy. There's a good chance your body will respond by going into starvation metabolism, and there's an even better chance you'll put back on any lost weight as soon as you come off the diet.

Forget about magic food theories. They're myths made popular by magazines trying to sell copies at the grocery store checkout.

Weighty Warning _____

There are ways to help your body burn food faster, but grapefruit isn't it. No single food can do it. But you can "inspire" your body to burn food faster by increasing your metabolism through strength training and aerobic exercise, reducing stress, and avoiding starvation metabolism. An extra caution about grapefruit: Grapefruit juice can interfere with certain prescription medications such as statins, which are cholesterol-lowering medications, beta-blockers, and calcium channel blockers.

Low-Fat Diets

Is fat the enemy? Many low-fat diets recommend that you reduce fat to 10 percent or less of your total caloric intake to make your heart healthier. This may not be enough fat for you to lose weight and have good health. The low-fat diets either don't recommend or ignore altogether the essential fatty acids that assist with weight loss and improve heart health. They advocate eating low-fat processed foods that are filled with sugars and high-glycemic starches. Recent studies show that eating high–glycemic starches, such as French bread, bagels, and cookies will increase your LDL, low-density lipoproteins, (the bad cholesterol) levels. Extreme low-fat diets are not a good path to life-long thinness.

Yes, it is important to eat less dietary fat. However, avoid relying on an extreme low-fat eating plan. Its recommendations are not nutritionally sound and can be harmful. You can have a healthy heart without excessive restrictions on your eating.

Many low-fat diets fail to recommend consuming essential fatty acids, and many promote eating high-glycemic carbohydrates. You need essential fatty acids to keep your heart healthy, and the high-glycemic starches raise LDL cholesterol levels, contributing to heart disease.

Thinspiration

Even with the push from the medical community and the American Heart Association to reduce the amount of dietary fats eaten, Americans are eating more fat than ever before. In 1942, the average American ate 42 pounds of fat annually. Today, on average, we eat 60 pounds.

Does this suggest we should commit ourselves to buying and eating only food labeled "low fat"? Absolutely not. In 1942, low-fat processed foods didn't exist. Yet overweight rates were much lower, under 28 percent of the population. Today, about 65 percent of the U.S. population is classified as overweight or obese.

What's gone wrong? Should we stop eating fat? If ever there was a universally declared "evil food," it's fat. The fear of fat has spawned an entire category of grocery store foods labeled "low fat" that haven't helped us get thinner as a population.

The crux of the problem isn't eating fat; rather, it's overeating fat. The average American eats from 39 to 50 percent fat in his or her diet. That's too much. It makes sense to reduce this to between 20 and 30 percent. You don't need to eat less than that.

You don't need to eat only low-fat foods to keep the percentage of fat in your diet in line with reasonable guidelines. Many of us get too much fat, not because the foods we eat contain fat but because the portions we eat are too large. A healthy diet can include some French fries, but a "supersize" order of fast-food fries is asking for trouble.

If you cut down the quantity of food you eat overall, you'll automatically reduce the amount of fat you're eating. Do this by only eating when your stomach is hungry and stop eating when you are satisfied, before you feel full. This is called eating 0-5. More information about this is in Chapter 5.

Zone Eating

The basic premise of the "zone" eating program is to eat about 40 percent carbohydrates, 30 percent protein, and 30 percent fat on a daily basis. This is excellent. So far, so good. But there's no reason why you will lose weight eating this way unless you also only eat when hungry and stop before you're full.

Among the food recommendations, some foods, such as eggs, are tagged as bad for you. We don't agree with this.

Eating the specific nutrient ratios, give or take, can be done over a lifetime.

Packaged foods for zone eating are now available. The ingredients are healthful, and we love that the foods don't need to be frozen or refrigerated, so they could be convenient for traveling. Remember to use packaged foods as a convenience item, eating them once in a while but not every day. Packaged foods do not contain your daily five fresh fruits and vegetables, so be sure to eat them in addition to a prepackaged convenience meal.

Overall, zone eating is fine. Make sure you also eat 0 to 5 to lose weight.

The No-Sugar Way

These diets recommend that a person avoid high-glycemic starches and sugars and instead limit carbohydrate intake to fruits and vegetables. Believers cite studies showing that high-glycemic carbohydrates stimulate the body to overproduce insulin, thus prompting fat storage. Usually these diets offer balanced eating, with a recommendation of 30 percent proteins, 30 percent fats, and 40 percent carbohydrates. So far, we agree that this is a good and healthy way of eating.

But then some of the no-sugar diets get off track. Some recommend aspartame or saccharine as sugar substitutes. Please don't use these at all. Some no-sugar plans may recommend food combining, which you can totally ignore. Some of the plans may suggest that you are allowed one day or one meal a week to eat anything you want. We abhor this idea. A binge day is not healthy or good common sense. In fact, it encourages a person to overeat and to harm his or her body.

While we support the premise of reducing sugars and starches, we don't like the rigidity and strict rules. Maintenance is difficult when the rules don't allow for eating a piece of wedding cake or a burrito. If you relax the rules to allow yourself to eat some high-glycemic starches as a condiment and you stay away from artificial sweeteners, you could find that these programs work for a lifetime.

> **CAUTION**
>
> **Weighty Warning**
>
> Beware of any diet systems that highly recommend that you eat artificial foods such as artificial sweeteners, preservatives, and colorings. Growing evidence suggests that these may be harmful to your health.

Diet in a Box

Many diet systems offer packaged foods that are available in the grocery store, discount stores, and on the Internet. The same criteria apply to these foods as to any others. Read the labels.

- Do they contain artificial ingredients?
- Are they low fat?
- Do they want you to substitute soy protein for meat, poultry, and fish?

◆ Are they full of sodium and salt?

◆ Do they contain high-glycemic carbohydrates?

If the answer to any of these questions is "yes," consider other alternatives. Just buy regular food and eat 0 to 5.

Other Specialty Diet Systems

The boxed cereal diet, the Subway diet, the shakes diet, the bread diet, and the cabbage soup diet are just a few of the funky diets that have made the rounds. Before the next millennium arrives, probably every food ever known to man will become a special "magical" way to lose weight! And all of them will probably work for somebody.

Even the weirdest diets can work, not because of the magic of the food or product but because the dieter makes them work. More likely than not, however, the systems won't work for the long term. They aren't nutritionally balanced, and some recommend ingredients that don't support your health.

So beware. Read the labels. Do your homework. If an eating approach doesn't feature a balanced diet, it's not going to work for the long term. In other words, make sure your diet contains a good-size serving of common sense before anything else.

The Least You Need to Know

◆ High-protein, low-carbohydrate diet plans can work short term, but without plenty of fresh fruits and vegetables, these plans fall short of good nutrition.

◆ Because your body needs fat (especially essential fatty acids) to release fat stores, eating a low-fat diet can actually inhibit weight loss.

◆ Specialty eating plans as a whole are seldom nutritionally balanced and may not deliver lifelong weight management.

◆ No special food exists that can cause weight loss or prevent weight gain.

◆ What works for long-term, lifelong weight loss is *you* and not any special system.

Medical Approaches to Weight Loss

In This Chapter

- Risks and rewards of weight-loss drugs
- Liposuction and tummy tucks
- Stomach surgery to control eating

Hasn't everyone who is overweight wished for the perfect little pill? The one that would melt away the fat virtually overnight? Of course. Has there ever been one? Yes and no.

The medical profession and pharmaceutical companies have been searching for "fat fixes" for many years. They know that solving our overeating problems with a pill would help lots of us improve our health, make us happier … and make *them* a lot of money. They keep trying.

Or maybe doctors can just make our stomachs smaller so that we have less urge to eat. Actually, they can.

Let's take a closer look at how the medical profession is tackling the weight problem.

The Search for the Perfect Pill

In the 1950s, there were amphetamines. Diet pills. Speed. They worked pretty well. They hyped a person up enough to burn calories. Eventually, we learned that they also ruined a person's health. They were highly addictive. They weren't safe. The FDA pulled them off the market.

Then, in the 1990s, another diet pill was formulated that produced great results for many people. Fen-phen soothed its users, and they no longer wanted to overeat. They lost weight almost effortlessly. Unfortunately, within a couple of years, several of them were dead. Fen-phen silently was causing pulmonary hypertension leading to lung and heart damage. This combination of pills wasn't safe. The FDA pulled them off the market.

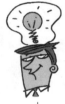

> **Thinspiration**
>
> Before you commit your body to prescription drugs for weight loss, ask yourself a simple question: "Why am I doing this?" If you think a pill will allow you to eat as much as you want, you're likely to be disappointed. Don't give up on the idea that you can adjust your eating and exercise habits to reach your ideal size naturally. Have confidence in your ability to master your size and your eating.

The search for the perfect prescription diet pill by the major drug companies goes on. Weight loss is big business, and the pharmaceutical industry is eager to find a successful diet pill.

Researchers are now exploring genetic coding and are actually looking for a way to alter a person's biology to prevent the body from storing fat.

> **Weighty Warning**
>
> All prescription drugs for weight loss bring with them serious side effects. Make sure you know all of them before you make your decision. Also, be sure to learn the average weight loss of users and how quickly users regain their weight when they go off the drug.

Even though obesity and being overweight have been declared a health epidemic, these conditions aren't caused by a bacteria or virus like other epidemics. Our collective chubbiness is caused by a lack of regular exercise, overeating, and poor food choices. Medical science may be better suited to finding vaccines for bacterial or viral infections. Solving a condition brought on by lifestyle decisions isn't an easy fit with the world of drugs. Yet the search goes on.

Here is information on some of the current drugs used for weight loss. They are only recommended for people who are obese, meaning they have a BMI equal to or greater than 30. If you are considering a weight-loss drug, keep these two questions in mind:

◆ What are the side effects, and can I live with them?

◆ What are the chances I will regain my weight?

Here's what is available by prescription.

Meridia

This pharmaceutical is also known as Reducil, and the common name is sibutramine. It is an appetite suppressant that is intended to be used with a low-calorie diet and exercise program. It stimulates various appetite-control centers in the brain and affect levels of brain neurotransmitters, which also can reduce appetite. It costs about $85 a month and is seldom covered by insurance. (Costs can vary considerably.)

Sibutramine has been deemed safe for only one year of use. You can expect to keep your weight off for up to a year. It's only recommended for people with a BMI of 30 or higher or for those with a BMI higher than 27 who are at risk for diabetes, high blood pressure, or high cholesterol.

Unwanted side effects can include raised heart rates and higher blood pressure. Sales of Reducil have been suspended in Italy after 50 reports of adverse reactions and 2 deaths. Overall, reports suggest that 34 deaths have been associated with taking this drug.

Body of Knowledge
All weight-loss drugs come with recommendations that include using a low-calorie diet and an exercise program. Even with medication, a person still needs to limit food intake and exercise regularly. Keep that in mind if you are considering using medications for weight loss.

Xenical

Also called Orlistat, this drug is used for the treatment of chronic obesity. It reduces your body's ability to absorb fat from the foods you eat. In essence, it is a fat blocker. It works best if you are able to stick to a low-calorie diet and a regular exercise regime.

The side effects include gas, increased frequency of bowel movements, and fatty/oily stool. We have heard of people who "leak," so to speak, while on this drug. This is also called fecal incontinence.

Since your body needs fat, especially essential fatty acids, we hate to think that users miss the benefits from the fats they eat. Bottom line, this drug is unpleasant.

Clinical trials show it's safe for up to two years of use.

Phentermine

This half of the banned fen-phen weight-loss pill is still approved for use. Also called Adipex, Phentermine is an appetite suppressant that is similar in molecular structure to amphetamines. It is habit forming. Phentermine increases your heart rate and blood pressure and decreases your appetite. Because it is chemically similar to amphetamines, a person could become addicted to this drug.

Needless to say, a person can't stay on phentermine for a lifetime. The likelihood of regaining your weight once you stop taking this drug is extremely high.

Other Drug Possibilities

Some medications that have been approved by the FDA for other medical conditions are now being considered for use as weight-loss drugs. The following show promise:

- ◆ Wellbutrin is an antidepressant. People using it may experience small weight loss.
- ◆ Topamax is an antiepilepsy drug. It has been shown to suppress appetite but can have serious side effects.
- ◆ Glucophage is a diabetic drug that improves sensitivity to insulin. It may prevent weight gain and make a diet program more effective, but it can also have serious side effects.

Lean Lingo

Liposuction is a surgical process in which fat is suctioned from the areas of your body where excess amounts are stored. A plastic surgeon will make one or more small incisions through your skin layers and then suction out the fat cells. The procedure is usually performed in a doctor's office or clinic rather than a hospital.

Fat Removal ... Literally

Perhaps you have thought that rather than trim the amount of food you eat, you could just pay a surgeon to trim the fat out of your body. We're talking about liposuction, tummy tucks, and other surgical fat-removal techniques.

Liposuction and tummy tucks certainly can take away the fat. The surgeon cuts it out or siphons it out. When you come out of surgery, you will have thinner thighs, a smaller derriere, or a flatter tummy. These days, plastic surgery isn't just limited to below the waist. People are having their upper arms, waists, breasts, and other body places liposuctioned.

If you've inherited saddlebags that no amount of exercise or diet will reduce, liposuction could be a choice. But we need to tell you that those saddlebags can grow back even after liposuction. Body fat tends to be stored in the same places as before surgery. Several girlfriends have had their thighs done more than once.

Is liposuction or a tummy tuck for you? Only you and your bank account know the answer to that question. They're definitely *not* long-term answers to your weight problems. A surgeon can't cut out your poor eating habits. The weight will come right back if you overeat. So approach surgery knowing that your long-term success depends on eating as a thin person for the rest of your life.

> **Weighty Warning**
>
> Liposuction is not a weight-loss solution. Rather, it's an expensive cosmetic surgical process to reshape unwanted bulges and fat areas. Without balanced eating and exercise throughout your lifetime after surgery, you will regain the fat areas that the liposuction got rid of.

Liposuction is serious surgery. It requires anesthetics and can have complications. Make sure you find a surgeon who is board certified and get recommendations from your regular doctor. Good plastic surgeons want you to be at your ideal weight *before* they operate so that they can take away the saddlebags you were, in essence, born with.

Plastic surgery is expensive and is not covered by health insurance. Expect to pay several thousand dollars for a surgeon to rid you of saddlebags or give you a flat tummy.

Stomach Surgery

This is serious stuff. Don't even think of this drastic step unless you have a BMI of 40 or above. The operation, commonly referred to as "stomach stapling," is called gastric bypass or bariatric surgery. The surgery is not a guarantee that you won't regain your weight. We have participants in our weight-loss classes who have had their stomachs stapled. Some of them are still paying off the loans for their surgery, yet they're back in class to lose weight.

The Roux-en-Y is abdominal surgery in which the stomach is stapled to a lower area in the small intestine—bypassing approximately 155 centimeters of small intestine. Problems with this surgery include increased complications of leaking at the bypass sites, significant and persistent diarrhea, and a mortality rate of about 1.5 percent. About 20 percent need additional surgery to remedy complications and 30 percent develop nutritional deficiencies.

Body of Knowledge

Stomach surgery is a booming business. The American Society for Bariatric Surgery estimates that the number of weight-loss surgeries in 2002 will be about 62,400, which is over three times the number performed five years ago.

The adjustable gastric band is a new and reportedly safer and easier form of stomach surgery. The adjustable gastric band (or the abdominal band, as it is sometimes called) has been more popular in Europe, although it is now being used in the United States. It is safer then Roux-en-y surgery, which until now has been more commonly used in the United States. People lose two to three pounds per week over the first year and then usually maintain weight after that.

The adjustable gastric band is installed laparoscopically through small incisions in the abdomen rather than through a major incision. Essentially, the band clamps around the stomach to limit the amount of food you can get into it. A valve is inserted in the chest area, and the doctor can use it to tighten or loosen the band.

Even after stomach surgery, you must make a lifetime commitment to exercise and diet to stay at your ideal size. Because this is really serious surgery, be prepared to handle complications and side issues. Some people find the surgery to be a dream come true. They have much less appetite and few side effects. Others have trouble eating even simple foods and risk an increased problem of vomiting with meals. No one can predict your outcome. Before you downsize your stomach, learn everything you can about the process and talk to others who have had the surgery.

While there are exceptions, don't expect this surgery to be covered by your health insurance.

The Least You Need to Know

♦ Prescription drugs for weight loss have a track record of serious side effects and seldom solve lifetime weight-loss issues.

♦ Consider using diet pills only if your BMI is 30 or above and you and your doctor agree that you must lose weight for health reasons.

♦ Cosmetic surgery, such as liposuction, is not intended for weight loss but rather to reshape the body.

♦ Bariatric or gastric bypass surgery is major surgery that can have serious complications; it should be considered only by the seriously obese whose BMI is 40 or above.

Chapter 24

Alternative Weight-Loss Choices

In This Chapter

- ◆ Pills, potions, and herbs
- ◆ Wraps, coaching, and hypnosis
- ◆ Ending the scams

Alternative choices for weight loss are plentiful. Weight-loss products that are supplements aren't regulated under the same requirements as prescription drugs. Many are good choices; many are scams. Before you leap into using an alternative choice, make sure you read the fine print and ask for proof of long-term success or a money-back guarantee.

Pills and Potions

You see the ads everywhere—in the newspaper, on late-night TV, in magazines, and on street corner posters. Your friends are selling weight-loss supplements. So is your doctor. The aisles in drug stores, health-food stores, and discount stores are well stocked with weight-loss formulations. It is impossible to escape the barrage of products that supposedly will make you thin once and for all. Or will they?

CAUTION

Weighty Warning _____

Do all those weight-loss ads sound too good to be true? They are. Read the small print. Somewhere on the page with the glamorous before-and-after pictures, the copy reads, "Results shown are not typical." Before you buy, ask for the company's documented research for what is the average weight loss. You'll likely be surprised at how little weight the average person loses.

Advertising claims for weight loss tell how much weight or how many inches a person lost in a specific time range. Much more pertinent information that isn't included is how long the person kept the weight off and how he or she maintained the loss. In other words, what's important to know is, where are the models today and how do they look?

Herbal Supplements

Herbal supplements for weight loss work by increasing your resting metabolic rate and by lifting your moods. These products are not monitored by the Food and Drug Administration. The safety of these herbal combinations may or may not have been tested by the product manufacturer. Most often the products are pills, but they can also be skin patches.

Ephedra combined with caffeine is the herbal concoction used in many weight-loss supplements. Often the caffeine comes from an ingredient such as guarana, green tea, or kola nut. The ephedra may be listed in the ingredients as ma huang or country mallow.

The weight-loss results from taking these products are attributed to the amphetamine-like effects of the combination of ephedra and caffeine. This combination may increase blood pressure and heart rate, thus causing the body metabolic rate to increase. They work on the nervous system pathway of the body through the adrenal glands. The herbs often reduce appetite and make a person feel energized.

Lean Lingo _____

Ephedra comes from a shrub-like plant found in desert areas throughout China and Mongolia and has been used medicinally for over 2,000 years. Its active ingredients are the alkaloids ephedrine and pseudoephedrine. Diet products contain concentrated extracts of ephedra.

As you might guess, the pills hype you up. Many people lose weight quickly without having to monitor their food intake and without exercise. These formulations seem to increase muscle mass because the body fat stores are used for energy. But does it last? When you stop taking the pills, you typically regain any weight you've lost and often even more weight. The weight gain tends to be fat, so a person can appear pudgy or bloated.

While taking an ephedra-based supplement, if you also develop the habit of eating balanced meals from 0 to 5 on the hunger scale and exercising regularly, you may be able to taper off ephedra and still maintain some of the weight loss. But there are other health reasons to consider different alternatives.

Ephedra is a powerful but risky supplement. The safety of ephedra combined with caffeine is embroiled in an ongoing controversy. Several deaths have resulted from using these types of diet pills, and there are many reports of strokes. Less severe side effects include increased anxiety and sleeplessness. These pills should not be used by persons with anxiety disorders, glaucoma, thyroid disease, diabetes, heart disease, or high blood pressure or anyone who takes monoamine oxidase (MAO) inhibitor drugs.

A second herbal combination for fat burning has recently been developed that does not use ephedra. Instead, the ingredients are *bitter orange*, also called citrus aurantium, in combination with caffeine. This combo gives a gentler lift in metabolism and somewhat slower weight-loss results.

The active ingredient in bitter orange is synephrine, which also has amphetamine-like effects. As of this writing, bitter orange is generally regarded as safe. What isn't known is how the body will react to ingesting the concentrated extract of bitter orange several times daily for long periods of time, nor have studies been conducted regarding the safety of its long-term use for weight loss. We also don't know if people can easily keep their weight off after they stop using products containing it.

Herbal weight-loss supplements are seldom the best answer for long-term, safe weight loss. They can sometimes produce short-term results, but they can't take the place of balanced eating, eating 0 to 5, and regular exercise.

Popular herbal weight-loss products that use the preceding ingredients are Metabolife, Herbalife, and HydroxyCut. The one- or two-page full-color ads for weight-loss supplements in magazines are most likely touting products that contain either ephedra or bitter orange.

Lean Lingo

The **bitter orange** in over-the-counter diet pills is also known as citrus aurantium or Seville oranges. This is the kind of orange used to make orange marmalade. Its active ingredient, synephrine, has mild amphetamine-like stimulant qualities.

Bedtime Formulations

If only you could shed extra pounds in your sleep. Some products claim you can. The user takes a spoonful or two of a substance right before bed, and the pounds supposedly melt away.

The catch is this: You can't eat any food for three hours before bedtime. Obviously, this would help many people lose weight because overweight people often consume a lot of food during the evening hours before bed. So if someone normally turns in around 10 P.M., you can bet he or she will lose some weight just by refraining from eating anything after 7 P.M. Hardly a miracle diet pill. The person's weight loss, if there is any, may result from consuming less food and not from consuming a pill or potion.

The ads claim amazing weight-loss results. There are no recommendations for balanced eating or exercise. A scientist from one of the companies stated on a popular television show that the average weight loss by consumers was half a pound. Wow, huh? Pass on bedtime weight potions.

Product names include Calorad and Body Solutions.

Body Wraps

Guess what? Your body contains a lot of water, and water weighs a lot. Maybe the solution to losing weight is as simple as sweating away your body's water. Well, it works! It's also the most temporary, expensive, and silly way to try to lose weight.

Imagine going to a lovely salon and having your entire body wrapped so that you sweat a lot—a whole lot. Your hands and feet are covered with plastic bags. During the next hour, you sit in a steam room, perhaps even exercise. When you are unwrapped—voilà!—you have miraculously lost 10 to 12 pounds and some inches off your waist! Strike up the band!

But wait! What happens if you drink some water and eat a meal? Surprise! Back comes the water weight. And chances are good you'll want to drink lots of water because your body naturally craves it. It wants to be replenished.

We get a chuckle that the advertising for body wraps only promises "semipermanent weight loss." Now that's an understatement! These weight-loss sweat systems are expensive and obviously are not

Thinspiration

If sweating is your thing, skip the body wrap and do some really serious exercising. Climb a mountain. Play racquetball. Get on the bike. That way, you're actively burning off stored fat and boosting your metabolism, too. The key to the success of this type of activity isn't the sweating; it's the muscular exertion and aerobic effect that make the real positive impact.

long-term solutions. Recent complications include serious skin infections and systemic infections. We're not aware of scientific studies about their safety.

One-on-One Coaching

If you're at your wits end and don't know where to turn or what to do to get the weight off, consider using a weight-loss coach or a registered dietitian. He or she can help you make sense of your weight-loss issues and can help you determine what will work best for you.

A weight-loss coach can give you a doable food and eating plan, a practical exercise plan, an accountability system, emotional support, a feedback system so you can make changes if the program needs adjusting, and suggestions for supplementation. When interviewing weight-loss coaches, be sure the coach doesn't insist that the only way to lose weight is by taking weight-loss products he or she sells. Use a coach who is already at his or her ideal size, make sure the coach has appropriate credentials or a great track record, and make sure he or she recommends supplements only to support a healthy, balanced weight-loss program.

To ensure your success when working with a weight-loss coach, be sure to tell all. Yes, even about the two drinks you have every evening or how quickly you get to the bottom of ice cream cartons. Francie was a sweet single woman who kept trying to lose some stubborn weight. One day, she calmly confessed that maybe, just maybe, the munchies she got from smoking pot every night before bed might be part of her problem!

Yes, a coach needs to know everything that's relevant. If you can't divulge your little eating secrets, don't waste your time and money.

> ## Body of Knowledge
>
> Weight-loss coaches are not all the same. For instance, one may emphasize detailed eating plans but may not give you tips to tackle the emotional issues surrounding your weight. Another may help you with a broader approach to weight loss by redirecting your eating habits. Investigate your coach before selecting him or her. Check out references and referrals.

Hypnosis

We give hypnosis mixed reviews. It works well for some people and not for others. Weight loss is not easily tackled by hypnosis. The problem is the nature of eating. Because we all need to eat, the hypnotist can't use an all-or-nothing approach, which works well for phobias and for smoking cessation.

If you want to try hypnosis, try to have an open mind but don't count on it working. As with any professional service, check out the hypnotist's credentials and check references.

Amazing Offers

They come up every day among the morning's e-mails. We get at least one sincerely written offer every day to buy a miraculous weight-loss product. We bet you get them, too. Occasionally, we read them to see what the latest promise is, but generally they go into that wonderful electronic trash bin where they belong. (We especially enjoy the messages that ask us to send cash only, no credit cards. Sound a little suspicious?)

The claims are on TV—especially on late-night TV. Maybe they've concluded that we're all more gullible then. All you have to do is phone their 800 number right away, and you, too, can be thin forever. We wish it were true. You know it's not. It's a gimmick, perhaps even a scam. Legitimate weight-loss systems offer scientific proof and, usually, money-back guarantees.

A special bread. A new type of pill. A new system. The claims will never stop, but they're very unlikely to work—and you don't know if they're safe or not.

Please don't spend your money on these scams. Instead, use good common sense. Eat a balanced diet, eat 0 to 5, and get plenty of exercise. Then use all that money for new clothes and vacations and other delightful luxuries. Or save it.

The Least You Need to Know

- Many alternative weight-loss programs are available, but few offer long-term weight loss.

- Supplements for weight loss almost always include herbs that cause amphetamine-type effects on blood pressure, heart rate, and anxiety.

- Beware of Internet and infomercial weight-loss scams that promote miraculous results.

- Working with a weight-loss coach or registered dietitian can help you develop a program that is right for you.

Part

Get Your Mindset Right

As you lose weight, you will emerge from your fat "skin" with your body transformed into your ideal size. In this part of the book, we show you how to greet the world as a thin person.

By adopting the mindset of being thin, you'll say goodbye forever to your fat self. You'll part ways with your fat thoughts, emotions, and behaviors.

You'll order from restaurant menus with confidence and enjoy celebrations and parties with grace and ease. You'll surround yourself with a support group to help you solidify your progress. You'll create a formal "Moving Beyond" exercise to emerge from your fat cocoon into a joyous, vibrant, and compassionate thinner person.

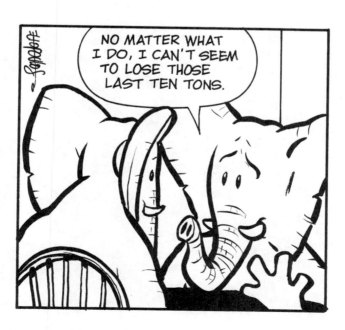

25

Think Yourself Thin

In This Chapter

- ◆ Using mental power
- ◆ Having clear intentions
- ◆ Being in charge
- ◆ Dealing with naysayers

Can you get to your ideal size by just thinking so? Yes, you can. We know people who have done it. You can give up having a weight issue. Just walk away from it. Adopt the attitude of "been there, done that." Convince yourself that you are already at your ideal size. How can you do this? By using your mental and emotional resources to make it so. Notice we didn't say to use willpower and self-discipline. By now you have enough experience with weight loss to know these don't work, so let's take a different approach. We suspect it is one you haven't tried before.

Believing Is Seeing

Never underestimate the power of your mental outlook. Researchers tell us that the brain doesn't distinguish between what you imagine and what is real. Yes, if you imagine that you are at your ideal size, your subconscious doesn't know if it is fact or fiction. The more you imagine and the more you turn away conflicting thoughts, the closer you get to being effortlessly thin.

People who are walking around on this planet in thin bodies do not think they are fat. They don't worry about what to eat, when to diet, or how to diet. The thoughts wouldn't cross their minds. Do the same for yourself. Here's how.

Cut Excuses Out of Your Thought Menu

You and only you are totally responsible for the size of your body. It wasn't the advertising that put the food into your mouth. It wasn't the stress either. It was only one thing—you. We want you to stop using excuses and take full responsibility for the size of your body. This action empowers you to make the changes necessary to get to your ideal size.

Yes, we mean that mom and the kids and the spouse and the hormones and on and on are not the real reason you have a weight issue. It was solely how you reacted to your life situations. For example, when Lucy got over the fact that her son had learning disabilities and that she had to deal with the situation rather than eat over it, she was finally able to release the fat. We know this sounds really tough and a bit ruthless, but we also know you want to be your ideal size.

You are in charge. Act in charge of your eating. Be picky and be impolite. After all, it is your body and not anyone else's. You have our permission to be obnoxious if necessary to avoid eating what you don't want or need.

Thinspiration

Learning to eat as if you were already thin can be fun. Take your thin friends out to lunch or dinner and observe how they eat. Then model their healthy eating behaviors, such as being picky eaters and not cleaning their plates.

If you find yourself wanting to make excuses for your size, stop mid word (just like you would stop mid bite if you were done eating). Then take it back, rephrase it, and say it in such a way that you are responsible and in charge. For example, if you say or even think, "I feel fat today," reword it and instead say aloud, "I feel thin today." Turning around your thoughts like this gives you power.

Forgiveness as Weight Loss Aid

Perhaps you started gaining weight from the stress of a major—or even minor—life event. Such things as divorce or loss of a loved one can trigger overeating for consolation. So can getting older and feeling older.

If you can release the trauma and sadness from such events and the people associated with them, you can often come to terms with overeating. To do this, use the power of forgiveness. In virtually every religion in the world, forgiveness is considered to be a highly sacred and spiritual practice. We agree.

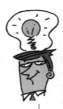 **Thinspiration**

Forgiveness is the act of pardoning without harboring grievances. The key to success with forgiveness is persistence, tenacity, and desire.

We also know that forgiveness has great power to heal wounds and release weight. So, if you feel burdened by past life events, as if you are still carrying around their weight, do your forgivenesses.

First make a list of everyone who was involved in your weight issue. Be sure to include yourself. Then make up some forgivenesses and write them down. Use the formula, "I, *(fill in your name)*, forgive you for *(whatever the issue)*. Also write forgivenesses for yourself, such as, "I, *(fill in your name)*, forgive myself for *(whatever the issue)*.

For yourself, you could write the following:

> I forgive myself for overeating.
> I forgive myself for getting older.
> I forgive myself for being overweight.
> I forgive myself for abusing my body with too much food.
> I forgive myself for not exercising.

One client came back to class the next week having begun the forgiveness homework exercise. She told the class that she had written 27 pages of forgivenesses, and she still wasn't finished forgiving her mother. But she said it was really a great feeling.

While it may sound somewhat shallow to forgive a person so that you can lose weight, well, if you haven't forgiven them already, perhaps it is time to do so. And the weight situation may be a treasured opportunity to let go of past grievances.

We figure it doesn't matter why you forgive. It just matters that you forgive.

Tell the Truth

Tell the real truth to yourself with compassion about what you eat, how much you eat, when you eat, and if you ate above a 5 or started eating above 0. We have clients who fudge when they record their hunger numbers. Now, just who are they cheating and why? Are they trying to look good to themselves?

We suggest that you use the form that follows to record your hunger numbers and food intake every day, for every meal, every snack, and every nibble. Record everything you put into your mouth except water. Be ruthlessly honest with yourself. That way, you get excellent results. You get the results you want.

Date: _____				
Time	Beginning Hunger #	Item	Amount	Ending Hunger #

So a typical meal could look this way:

Date: 02/02/02				
Time	Beginning Hunger #	Item	Amount	Ending Hunger #
8:35 A.M.	0	salmon	card deck size	
		green apple	small	5
6:15 P.M.	0	roast beef	card deck size	
		spinach salad	bowl	
		brownie	small	5
Percentage of day I was a thin person in mind and behavior = _____ %				

Notice that we don't want you to weigh and measure your food. We aren't asking you to weigh and measure your body, and we certainly aren't going to ask you to weigh and measure your food. Just record about how much it was. You know if it is too much food.

Record your food intake and hunger numbers every day until you are comfortably at your ideal size. You can continue as long as you want. If your jeans ever get tight, record your food intake and hunger numbers until they fit comfortably. We have done this off and on for over 20 years.

Ban Diet Paraphernalia

People who have the mindset of being thin do not keep diet stuff around the house. Let's say you didn't own a dog, never owned a dog, and didn't have any plans to have a dog. Yet you owned a dog dish, a leash, dog food, and purchased books on raising and breeding dogs. You would appear nuts.

Ditto believing you are thin. Thin people don't have freezers stocked full of diet and low-cal foods. They don't have large clothes in their closets just in case they regain their weight. All the clothes in their closets fit. They get rid of clothes because they are worn out, soiled, or out of style, not because they don't fit. They don't own dozens of books on weight-loss plans. If they did, they would seem nutty.

Thinspiration

Toss out anything in your refrigerator that you purchased with the hope that it would make you thinner. Get rid of low-fat salad dressings, low-fat ice cream and yogurt. Remember to get rid of fake butter and those "spreads" that are filled with trans fatty acids that are designed to taste like the real thing. And what about that low-fat cheese? Now go to the grocery store and buy real foods just like naturally thin people do.

Toss out your cache of diet paraphernalia. Give it away. Get it out of your sight. It will mess up your thin thinking to constantly see a food scale on the kitchen counter. Be consistent inside and out with being a thin person.

Ban Fat Thoughts

Stop telling yourself you are fat. Stop saying you are so big that .... Refuse to believe it even when the mirror says otherwise. Sometimes we are our own worst enemies when it comes to weight.

When Linda was overweight, she cried about it a lot and constantly talked about her problems with her weight, eating, and food. One day, as her husband was once again drying her tears, he said, "I think things would get a whole lot better for you if you would just stop telling yourself you're fat."

Linda, already wounded, said, "So what do you know?" Later she had to apologize when she realized he knew a whole lot.

> She stopped crying about her weight issue.
> She stopped talking about it.
> She stopped commiserating with her fat friends.
> She stopped buying diet foods.
> She stopped telling herself she was fat—and ugly.
> She stopped seeing food as the enemy.

She got in control of her eating, and she lost the weight down to her ideal size.

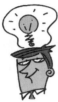

Thinspiration

Take one day and monitor your thoughts about your weight, eating, and size. You might be amazed at the sheer number of negative messages you send to yourself. These kinds of thought only reinforce your weight issue and make it more difficult to attain your ideal size.

How High Is Your Desire?

Ask yourself what percentage of the time you are willing to think and act as a thin person. How often are you willing to eat 0 to 5? How often will you eat sensuously and beautifully?

If your answer is about 50 percent of the time, your odds of success are less than 50 percent, more like about 5 percent. However, if you can give it your all, or 100 percent, for as long as it takes, you will definitely get to your ideal size.

But "as long as it takes" is sort of meaningless to schedule in your daily planner. So instead, ask yourself this question every day: "What percentage of my day was I a full participant in being a thin person?" If you had moments that were less than 100 percent, review each situation and ask yourself what you could have done better.

As long as you know deep in your heart that you are thinking and eating as a thin person every day, you absolutely know you will reach your goal.

When Suzie arrived at a luncheon date with a college friend way below 0, she could have eaten the proverbial horse, so to speak. Suzie dove into the white bread and then proceeded to eat all of her lasagna and salad. When she stood up to leave, she was between a 9 and a 10 on the hunger scale. Looking back on her experience, she could have ordered a glass of fruit juice when the waiter first came to the table and then sipped it slowly until her hunger level got up to 0. Then, when the entrée came, she would have had the ability to eat normally—that is, to eat from 0 to 5.

At the end of each day, ask yourself what percentage of the day you ate and thought as a thin person.

Thinspiration _____

Let your true desire fuel your weight-loss success. Wanting may not be the same as getting, but without the wanting, you most likely won't get. Build your desire and pave the way to your inner and outer success.

The Naysayers

You've met naysayers before. They are people who tell you it will never work, that they have tried that method before and it didn't work for them, so why should it work for you?

Beware the naysayers who notice that you are eating differently and try to break your resolve. Others will lecture you on how weight loss really works and will let you know that you are doing it all wrong. Some actually push food on you and insist you eat what they want you to eat.

Maria was obviously overweight and was enjoying an ice cream cone while sitting outside on a bench at popular neighborhood shopping area. A strange woman approached her, sat down next to her, and said, "Are you sure you should be eating that ice cream cone?" Then she proceeded to tell Maria that she had lost all sorts of weight recently and told her how she did it. Maria just got up and walked away. The nerve of some people. We would like to think that this strange woman had good intentions—but she sure didn't have good boundaries.

How do you handle these people, whether they are doing it for your own best good or not? First and foremost, don't tell anyone you are on a plan to lose weight. Even if people ask, don't tell them. If they notice you have lost weight and want to know how, refer them to this book. But it is best to avoid a long story and detailed description. Here are some suggestions for handling these pushy people:

Thinspiration _____

Build yourself a base of good support. First create the support within yourself and then find support in books, friends, and even on the Internet. Use this support when anyone challenges your goals and your weight-loss program.

- ◆ **The food pusher.** Say one of these two things: "Oh, no thanks, not right now, it looks delicious, but I'm saving room for dinner." Or say, "I'm just not hungry right now. It looks delicious, perhaps later."

- **The family member food pusher who wants you to eat more dessert or go back for seconds.** Put your hand across your tummy and say, "Thanks, your food was wonderful, but I just can't fit in another bite."

- **The "Are you sure you should be eating that?" person.** Answer "Absolutely!" and walk away.

- **The know-it-all-about-dieting person.** Say thanks but no thanks, especially if they aren't at their ideal size. It is best to learn from someone who has already mastered weight, not someone who is still trying to figure it out.

- **The fat friend.** This one is tough because it is possible you could lose some fat friends along the way if you master your weight. To stay friends, find other mutual interests.

- **Any potential naysayer.** The less you say, the less they can hurt you.

If you do happen to get in the path of a naysayer, as soon as you escape, be sure to repeat your inner mantra—see the following section —to yourself until any inner turmoil goes away and you get recentered as a thin person.

The Inner Mantra

Directing your thoughts to being thin is really hard. After all, you have years of scripts and self-talk that do anything but affirm your thin self. That's why we recommend you use the ideal size *affirmation*. This is the only one you need to use.

It goes like this, "I, (*insert first name*), am now a healthy and thin person. I wear a size (*insert desired size*), and I do what healthy and thin people do."

This statement affirms exactly what you want. If the word "thin" for you doesn't mean what it means to us, change it so that you are comfortable. Most often a person will change it to "lean." But we urge you not to change anything else. For example, don't change it to say, "I deserve to be thin." That is a lame and actually ineffective affirmation. Our response would be, "So what if you deserve to be thin? Deserving and being are two different things."

The secret of this affirmation is that it declares you are already there. Yes, you will be shaking things up in your mind. This is good. You will be creating cognitive dissonance in your mind. Since this makes you uncomfortable, your insides will work hard to bring about compliance with your affirmation. Getting to

Lean Lingo

An **affirmation** is a carefully written positive statement declaring that you already have what you want. It usually starts with the words "I am" and states in present tense your desire as if you already have it.

your ideal size will require less and less thought and effort. In fact, you will be amazed at how easy it is to eat 0 to 5 after a couple months of using the affirmation.

To use the affirmation, say it aloud at least three times in a row three times a day. Yes, you can say it in private. That's a great start. It works even faster if you write it. That's right, write the affirmation 10 times every day. Purchase a spiral notebook or a fancy journal and write the affirmation 10 times every day. Do it with meaning and care. At first, parts of your psyche will rebel. Let them. The writing will, over time, convince them that you are indeed a healthy and thin person.

If a situation comes up that challenges you, such as the desire to stress eat or if your favorite donuts show up at work and you aren't at 0, say your affirmation to yourself. Save the donut until you are once again at a 0.

Lucy continued to write her weight-loss affirmation for six months after she had reached her ideal size. She has stayed at her ideal size for over 20 years. The time spent was a terrific investment.

Affirmations are one of the strongest and most effective tools for achieving your ideal size. We know plenty of people for whom this has worked. We also know people who have met their life's soul mate, improved their vision, and found terrific jobs by using the power of affirmations.

In a sense, you already affirm every day all day long. You have been affirming that you have an overweight body for years. Now change the "CD" and get what you really want.

What Is Your Intention?

Getting to your ideal size once and for all changes your life in many ways. Make sure you are ready to live with the changes. They can be wonderful, and yet even wonderful changes can be unsettling and may take some time to get used to. To aid you in making those changes, you can use the following intention statements. These are very powerful and can let you make major changes in your weight and your life.

Thinspiration

Writing and saying the ideal size affirmation can quickly shift your overeating. When your subconscious knows it is already at your ideal size, you may find you are simply eating 0 to 5 without a whole lot of effort.

Thinspiration

Make these new ways of thinking a part of your daily life. Think about them, or say them to yourself during idle moments, such as when waiting for the elevator, waiting at a traffic light, or standing in line at the grocery store. You can't overdo them and repetition brings the rewards you desire.

◆ I am now a size _____ in body, mind, and spirit.

Getting to your ideal size just in your body without mental and spiritual alignment can make you gain your weight back really fast. When all aspects of you
are totally aligned with being and with staying at your ideal size, you will.

◆ I am happy, comfortable, and safe being at my ideal size.

For many people, feeling happy, comfortable, and safe at a smaller size can seem
impossible. They have built a fortress with their body for protection. Find real
ways that you can be happy, comfortable, and safe and not use your body as a
fortress.

◆ I honor my body and its messages.

This refers to all the body's messages: the need to eat, the need to stop eating,
the need for sleep, for relaxation, for exercise, and movement. You may have
been taught to ignore the body's signals as an indication of inner strength.
Now it's time to learn that a person can't be a good caretaker of the body by
ignoring it.

◆ I love, enjoy, and appreciate my body.

Perhaps as you were growing up, you were taught that the body is bad.
However, we figure that the body is how you get through this life. Without a
body, well, you wouldn't be here. We find that when people can love, enjoy, and
appreciate their bodies, often overeating as a subtle form of self abuse ends.
Most of our weight-loss clients are "body" people. They require lots of physical
activity—either passive or active—to feel good, to be creative, and to be happy.

◆ I honor all of my emotions and use them responsibly.

Rather than stuffing emotions with food, which is not using emotions responsibly, learn how to use and express them with love. Also, remember to lift your
moods with cardio/aerobic exercise to get the endorphin lift.

◆ I am in harmony with being at my ideal size.

Be sure that all of the aspects of you can function fully and excellently when you
are at your ideal size. If you have a tiny voice inside that is fearful or even
alarmed at the thought, talk with that part until you understand the fear and can
make changes so that all of you is in harmony.

◆ I honor my sexual energy and express it appropriately.

Sexual energy as we use it here is a fabulous life-force power that can be used to
enhance all of your life. It is not only about physical intimacy but rather sexual
energy in all its forms. Even if you do not have a spouse or lover, you are still

expressing sexual energy in how you work, walk, talk, and eat. No, we're not in any way talking about promiscuity. We are talking about being in the flow of joy, abundance, and love.

To start using these intentions, set aside some time. Then take each one in turn and say the intention to yourself. As resistance comes up, listen to your inner resistant reasons and then repeat the intention to yourself. Do this over and over again until you can feel in harmony or in congruence with each intention.

These intentions were carefully designed to include the biggest fears and resistances a person has about being at his or her ideal size. At the class session a week after we give these intentions as homework, the participants return looking radiant, as if years of weight gain have been lifted from their bodies (and for some of them, a dress size has been lifted also).

Using the power of your mind and doing some mental and spiritual work can magnify your weight-loss efforts. The mental and spiritual work is like a booster engine, accelerating your weight-loss progress and lightening up your life.

The Least You Need to Know

- Accessing the power of your mind through affirmations can greatly accelerate your weight-loss progress.

- When you totally own your weight issues as your own and take full responsibility for your eating by giving up excuses, you can make consistent progress.

- Use forgiveness to get beyond any emotional and spiritual barriers to being your ideal size.

- Use intentions to clear out any fears about being your ideal size and use them to steer your mind toward reaching your goal.

Chapter 26

Eat Out Fearlessly

In This Chapter

- ◆ Eating out with ease
- ◆ Knowing what to order
- ◆ Sharing meals, bringing home leftovers
- ◆ Finding a healthy choice in every cuisine

Imagine eating out at any kind of restaurant—fast food, gourmet dining, or an all-you-can-eat buffet—without thinking about dieting. Thin people don't think about dieting when they eat out. Why should you? Instead, eat like you're already at your ideal size!

Does this mean you can pig out? Of course not. When you're enjoying life at your ideal size, why would you ever pig out? It doesn't make sense.

So how do you eat out like someone at his or her ideal size? Actually, it's not hard. Every dining out opportunity can help you reach and stay at your ideal size, even as you thoroughly enjoy the tastes and pleasures of the food. In this chapter, we tell you how.

What Eating Out Is About

Twenty years ago, forecasters predicted that Americans would begin to eat out much more often. Boy, were they ever right! Why do we do it? For

Lean Lingo

To **dine** means to eat beautifully. Dining means thinking about your hunger number, giving thanks for your food, eating slowly, having a good time, and stopping eating when your stomach is comfortable. You can dine any time you eat out, even at fast-food restaurants. You can also, of course, dine at home.

starters, eating out is convenient. Our lives seem busier than ever before, and we prefer not to take time to purchase and prepare foods. Second, we like to be served. It's just plain nice to have someone else prepare and serve food to us. Finally, it's for pleasure. We eat out for new tastes, for superb dishes, for relaxation, as a treat, to get away from the house, and for all sorts of pleasurable reasons.

Plain old nourishment is the least important reason. This is a good thing, actually. When you're eating out, you want the camaraderie, the friendship, the family, and all the pleasures of the experience to be more important than just eating. The food certainly counts, but let it be only one part of your total enjoyment. Even in a fast-food restaurant, you can choose to *dine*, or you can eat to get the food down and be done with it.

But I Paid for It!

Herein lies the biggest eating-out problem for overweight people: They feel obliged to eat everything served. They think, "If I paid for it, you bet I'm going to eat it." They think that if they don't eat all of the food served, they're wasting money.

This thinking is terrifically fattening. The hunger scale of 0 to 5 goes out the window once the food arrives because, well, you've paid for it. Instead, the diner *consciously overeats* to avoid wasting money ... then blames overeating on the amount of food served! This is like raising your hand and saying, "Over here! I'll pay you to help me get fatter!" It's just crazy.

If you've tended to think this way, please forgive yourself and resolve to change. If you don't change your perspective, you'll won't be able to eat out and also reach your ideal size.

Here are some incredibly simple ways to improve your eating out style:

1. **Eat enough (that is, eat up to 5 on the hunger scale) and take the rest home.** Leftovers can be a real treat and can stretch your food dollars. Never be embarrassed to ask for a take-home box. It's a thin thing to do.

2. **Share your meal with a friend.** Couples can regularly share meals, and perhaps you can share a meal with some of your friends, too. The waitperson seldom bats an eyelash, even in the fanciest restaurant. Order an extra salad or side vegetable if you want. Sharing an entrée also makes it easier to save room in your stomach for dessert.

3. **Think of eating out as entertainment.** View the food as just part of the total experience. That way, if you have a great time and only eat part of your meal, you'll still get your money's worth.

4. **Leave food on your plate.** Convince yourself that it's "cool" and enlightened not to eat everything you are served. It certainly is more of a thin way of eating.

> **CAUTION**
>
> **Weighty Warning**
>
> Don't let the quantity of food served or the attitude of a waitperson determine how you eat. The people who own, operate, or work at a restaurant aren't responsible for your weight. Only you are. Make sure you're in charge when you eat out.

Be a Picky Eater

Be a picky eater in a restaurant, just as you would at home. Order exactly what you want prepared exactly as you want it. If your favorite salad dressing is olive oil and vinegar with blue cheese crumbles, ask for just that. If you want your meat rare, ask for it rare. Don't be shy. You're paying.

If the food doesn't meet your standards, don't eat it. If you want to send it back to the kitchen, do so. Heck, if you want a certain pasta dish without the pasta, the cook can probably figure it out. Be polite but steadfast. After all, it's your tummy, your waistline, and your money we're talking about here.

> **Thinspiration**
>
> Be a picky eater when you eat out. By focusing on quality, not quantity, you're putting the emphasis on taste, not bulk. The shift in focus will help you slow down and make the most of more modest amounts consumed.

Consume the Basics

In eating out, make sure you follow the new food pyramid suggested in Chapter 9. It shouldn't be hard, even in ethnic restaurants. Every culture of the world eats proteins, carbohydrates, and fats. You should be able to find combinations of the three basic food groups that work for your body.

In choosing a restaurant, ask yourself these three questions:

1. Is my stomach now at 0? If not, can I be at 0 by the time we eat? When you don't start at 0, it will be harder to lose weight and may prevent you from staying at your ideal size.

2. Can I get at least 15 grams of high-quality complete protein in my meal at this restaurant? Fifteen grams is a portion about the size of a deck of cards. You

should be able to eat at virtually any restaurant in the world, with the possible exception of vegetarian restaurants, and get enough high-quality complete protein. At one of our favorite noodle restaurants, we order extra meat for our salad or pasta so we get enough.

3. Can I get enough vegetables and fruits? This is usually easy at regular sit-down restaurants but is not so common at many fast-food restaurants. The good news: Some of them now offer either salads or salad bars.

Eating Breakfast Out

Breakfasts belong in a class by themselves. Your food selection is critical for daylong high energy. If you don't consume good fuel at breakfast, you can't expect to have a great day. Here's some advice for eating smart breakfasts out.

Lean Lingo

The word **breakfast** is derived the Middle English word *brek* (meaning "to break") plus *fast* from the old Norse word *fasta* (meaning "to fast"). Thus, when you eat your first meal of the day, you break your fast—no matter what time it is.

Fortunately, restaurant breakfast menus list foods with plenty of protein and usually some kind of fruit. Choose the high-quality protein foods (such as ham, Canadian bacon, and eggs) that will help you avoid the late-afternoon slumps that lead to overeating. Regular bacon is a marginally acceptable food because it is highly processed and filled with nitrates. That usually goes for pork products and turkey bacon, too.

Here are some of your better choices for restaurant breakfast food:

- Eggs with ham or steak
- Omelets
- Eggs benedict
- Fresh fruit or fresh-squeezed juice
- Bacon (marginally acceptable)

Poorer choices include:

- High-glycemic starches such as pancakes, muffins, bagels, scones, waffles, toast, English muffins, and donuts
- High-glycemic cereals, which is pretty much all of them with the exception of steel-cut oatmeal and barley
- Sausage

The poorer choices aren't "evil foods," but you should not rely on them as your breakfast staple. If you really want pancakes, however, order your eggs or meat and one or two small pancakes. Use real butter on them and thoroughly enjoy their taste.

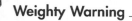

Weighty Warning

At a breakfast buffet, brunch, or other buffet-type meal, selectively choose what to put on your plate. Under no circumstances should you return to your table with a plate so loaded up that it looks like the foothills of the Rocky Mountains!

Breakfast buffets are challenging because of the variety and unusual food selections. You can become dazzled by the beautiful array of food and forget that your stomach is only about as big as your fist. An all-you-can-eat buffet is the perfect opportunity to practice your picky eating, enjoy the pleasures of eating beautifully, and not worry about maximizing how much food you're getting for your money. After all, why would you want to eat all that you can? It sounds fattening and uncomfortable.

So here's how to eat at a buffet. Even before you pick up your plate, walk around and check out the entire array of foods. Select which foods you definitely want to eat and which ones to pass on. If you see a dessert you really want, take it into account. As you go through the line with your plate, only put modest portions of the foods you really want.

Sit down, eat slowly, and enjoy your food. If the food doesn't taste as good as it looked, don't eat it. Eat up to 5. If you haven't reached 5, then and only then go back for seconds. You will be thrilled with this approach.

Best Bets for Lunch and Dinner

Three types of restaurants are usually quite reliable for eating out appropriately—that is, for getting enough protein, fruits, and vegetables.

Steak Houses

Steak houses abound in most cities and towns. Typically, the selection is focused on—you guessed it—steak. Sometimes seafood, too. You can easily make smart meal choices. Many offer salad bars or fabulous salads. If you make sure to eat 0 to 5, you can have a great meal that keeps you moving toward reaching your ideal size.

Best menu choices include:

- Steak or prime rib with visible fat cut off

- Seafood or fish

- Vegetable of the day

- Sautéed mushrooms

- Salad bar or salad

- Baked sweet potato with butter (these are moderate to low glycemic)

- Béarnaise sauce on veggies or meat

- Dessert of cheesecake or crème brûlée

Poorer choices include:

- White baked potato, especially if you plan to eat it all rather than just have a bite or two

- Anything starchy on the menu such as pasta

- Lots of bread

Since the size of the meals at steak houses can be large, they're a great place for sharing a meal. Or you can plan to bring leftovers home. That leftover steak makes a great and quick breakfast the next day.

Thinspiration

We include dessert recommendations because they can be an occasional special treat when eating out. Since many restaurants serve huge desserts, they're perfect for sharing if you're not yet at 5 on the hunger scale at the end of the meal. Remember that you can take home whatever is left over and sometimes eat a bite or two for several days. That's how we get our money's worth on desserts!

Hamburgers, Ribs, and Such

These are usually low- to mid-priced, sit-down restaurants. Example includes Bennigan's, Tony Roma's, and Chili's. They offer you wonderful choices for eating low glycemic and getting to your ideal size.

Best menu choices include:

- Burgers (hold the bun) and maybe a few fries

- Meat entrées such as chicken, ribs, and steaks

- Dinner salads and side salads

- Fish and seafood

- Ice cream for dessert (or another dessert that is low glycemic)

- Sandwiches—preferably hold the bread

Poorer choices include:

- Pasta dishes

- Sandwiches if you eat the bread

As you are beginning to notice, you can eat at any restaurant. Your food selections and eating 0 to 5 are what make you successful at getting to your ideal size.

Fresh Fish Houses

Any time you can eat fresh fish and seafood, go for it.

Good choices include:

- Fish and seafood entrées and appetizers

- Salads and veggies

- Butter, cocktail sauce, garlic sauce, or other condiments

Poorer choices include:

- Pasta dishes

- Too many French fries or too much baked potato

- Heavily breaded fish

- Sourdough bread (but if you can't resist the taste, limit your consumption to just a small piece)

> **Body of Knowledge**
>
> Because fish, especially salmon, contains essential fatty acids, most of us can benefit from eating more. Fish and other seafood are also excellent sources for quality protein.

Fast-Food Restaurants

Obviously, you don't go to a fast-food restaurant for gourmet dining (at least, we hope not!). But we assume you do end up at them every now and then. We do, too. They're convenient, inexpensive, and fast. You don't have to give up going to fast-food restaurants to reach your ideal size, but you do need to eat smart. For starters, ignore the "fast-food" label. Eat just as slowly as you do at other meals so that you taste the food, digest it well, and feel your hunger numbers—before, during, and afterward.

The Usual Drive-Thrus or Eat-Ins

Good choices at burger and chicken places include:

- Hamburger or cheeseburger (preferably toss the bun and eat the rest with a plastic fork)
- Salad
- Fried chicken (preferably remove the skin)
- Orange juice
- Mashed potatoes and gravy
- Coleslaw

Poorer choices include:

- French fries
- Milk shakes
- Diet sodas, colas, and pop
- Anything supersized (unless you are sharing with a whole Boy Scout troop or soccer team)

Delis and Sandwich Shops

These offer fast food with some more interesting choices. Subway has become an interesting place to eat. The company's commitment to informing customers about healthy eating, exercising, and getting to their best weight is to be applauded.

Good choices include:

◆ Whole-wheat wraps filled with meat, cheese, and lots of fresh veggies such as tomatoes, lettuce, cucumber, green peppers, and onions, as well as condiments such as black olives, pickles, and jalapeño chiles. You can open the wrap and eat the insides with a plastic fork. Yummy.

◆ A meatball sandwich with all the veggies and condiments. Eat with a fork, hold the bread.

◆ Any sandwich, hold the bread, with a couple of potato chips and a pickle.

◆ A piece of fresh fruit.

Poorer choices include:

◆ Eating all the bread on a sub (way too high glycemic!)

> **Weighty Warning**
>
> Sandwiches seem to be everywhere—at the ballpark, at athletic events, at picnics, and in box lunches. When you're trying to reach your ideal size, it sure helps to set aside all that bread. Don't worry about looking odd. With all the unusual ways people eat, few people will notice. Should a person be so impolite as to ask why you're not eating the bread, lightly shrug your shoulders and say, "I don't like bread." End of interaction.

Popular Specialty Eateries

Now let's talk about salad-bar restaurants and pizza parlors. Both are tricky to eat at healthfully and attain your ideal size.

Salad-Bar Restaurants

At these restaurants, you can choose from a wide offering of fresh fruits and vegetables that your body wants and needs. Plus, you get to select just exactly what you want to eat and how much. So what's not to like? The answer: the lack of enough high-quality complete protein.

Often you'll find sliced hard-boiled eggs and cheese, but salad bars seldom have meat or fish. You may find it a challenge to consume at least 15 grams of protein. You may be able to find some meat or seafood in a pasta salad, but you should generally pick out the meat and leave the white-flour pasta behind. Skip the high-glycemic pasta and baked potatoes you find these days.

Good choices include:

♦ Fresh fruits and vegetables

♦ Protein offerings such as hard-boiled eggs, cheese, and meat toppings

♦ Olive oil and vinegar dressing

Poorer choices include:

♦ Mayonnaise-based salads with pasta or potatoes

♦ Baked potatoes

♦ Pasta side dishes

♦ Starchy dessert offerings

♦ Loading up on salad dressing

♦ Low-fat salad dressings

CAUTION

Weighty Warning _____

Right now, picture your plate when you've been through the salad bar line. Does it look like a colorful mountain capped with enough salad dressing to ski down? Oops. Not good. Remember that your stomach doesn't need vast amounts of veggies and fruits to feel satisfied. Instead, eat just your favorites from the salad bar and return for more if you're not at 5 on the hunger scale.

Pizza

Pizza can be a big challenge when trying to reach your ideal size. It's the second most popular eating-out food behind burgers and for good reason—it smells great, it's a super treat, and it's easily served at everything from office luncheons to family parties. You even get to eat it with your fingers! Plus, it's only a quick phone call away. (P.S. Make sure the local delivery number isn't on your speed dialer!)

You'll never get away from pizza, and we don't want you to think of it as an evil food, but how you eat pizza can make a big difference in releasing fat from your body. Here are four pizza-eating tips:

First, when you get to choose the toppings, pick the meats or fish—ham, hamburger, anchovies, and Canadian bacon—and add veggies or fruits. Avoid ordering double cheese.

Second, when you eat pizza, eat with a fork. Eat the topping and leave behind the crust, no matter if the crust is deep dish or thin and crisp. Leave it for the trashcan. This will be a challenge, but give it a try.

Third, when you can, order a side salad with the pizza. You'll then have a fine and balanced meal that is low glycemic.

Fourth, eat slowly and make sure you eat 0 to 5. Don't even think about a third piece of pizza until you've stopped and checked with your body to see what your hunger number is.

Good choices include:

- Meat toppings (unfortunately pepperoni and sausage are the least desirable)
- Other vegetable and fruit toppings
- A side salad

Poorer choices include:

- Double cheese
- Highly processed meat toppings such as pepperoni and sausage
- The crust
- Eating pizza every day

If anyone has the insensitivity to ask you why you aren't eating the crust, just shrug your shoulders lightly and say, "The toppings are so good, I just don't want the crust." This should end the conversation, unless the person asks if he or she can eat your leftover crust.

Ethnic Food

Yes, you can eat comfortably at ethnic restaurants and enjoy the interesting, varied, and delightful cuisines. Remember to 1) consume the types of foods that best nourish your body, and 2) eat 0 to 5.

Mexican Food

Olé! Mexican and Tex-Mex cuisines are delicious, and if you enjoy spicy foods and hot chilies, these restaurants are hard to resist. Often high-quality complete protein comes wrapped in a starch—either corn or wheat tortillas or corn meal, as with tamales. Consequently, it's best to eat less of the wrapping and more of the filling. This is the same as our sandwich recommendations.

Good choices include:

- Guacamole dip
- Salsa with some corn chips
- Tortilla soup
- Carne adobada, or marinated long-cooked pork
- Carnitas
- Tamales, tacos, enchiladas, burritos, chimichangas, and other "wrapped" meat mixtures
- Salads
- Taco salad
- Fajitas
- Beans
- For dessert, flan (if you have room)

Thinspiration

If you really love the taste of the salsa that comes with the corn chips served before your meal at Mexican restaurants, it is fine to eat the salsa with a spoon and bypass all the chips. Salsa has great veggie value and great taste. It makes a great salad dressing, too!

Poorer choices include:

- Overeating the chips before the entrée arrives
- Eating all the rice or even most of it
- Ordering cheese rather than meat or chicken fillings
- Sopapillas for dessert (they're just fried bread)

You may find Mexican food so delightful that it's hard to stop eating at 5. Be sure to eat slowly so that you enjoy all the flavors; otherwise, it can seem as if 5 comes too soon.

Italian Restaurants

Even Italian food can help you get to your ideal size. Italian food isn't just pasta and breads; it includes fabulous meat and seafood dishes. Think veal piccata or scaloppini. Think fried calamari or mussels in a wine garlic sauce. Think fresh, sliced tomatoes with mozzarella and basil. Yes, you certainly can get a balanced meal and eat healthy at your favorite Italian eatery.

Good choices include:

◆ Beef, poultry, veal, fish, pork, and seafood entrées and appetizers

◆ Fresh salads such as Caesar and garden salads

◆ Small side dishes of pasta

◆ Fresh fruit, canolis, or cheesecake for dessert

◆ Extra meatballs with spaghetti

Poorer choices include:

◆ Pasta

◆ Fettuccine alfredo

◆ Eating more than a taste of bread

◆ Filling up on bread and pasta

Bring home what you can't eat. Meatballs make a great breakfast, as do other entrée choices.

Asian Restaurants

Asian cuisine is quite varied and, in this section, includes Chinese, Vietnamese, Korean, Thai, and others. The same fundamentals apply here as to eating out in general. Make sure you get enough protein and fresh fruits and vegetables.

Sometimes when you eat a dish that's stir-fried, it can be hard to judge if you've had enough protein. It's one reason why so many people feel hungry soon after eating oriental food. They seemed to eat plenty, but the food didn't contain enough high-quality protein to keep their engine stoked and their metabolism high.

Many Asian restaurants use MSG—monosodium glutamate—as a flavor enhancer for their food. We recommend that you always ask the waitperson to keep it out of your food.

Weighty Warning

Watch out for the huge portions served at Asian restaurants. Instead, stop when your stomach is comfortable before you are full and take the leftovers home, asking the waitperson to wrap the rice separately from the rest of the food. Or better yet, don't take the leftover rice home.

Good choices include:

- Meat-, fish-, and seafood-based dishes. (Make sure they contain more than just shreds of meat; they should have enough to make up an amount the size of a deck of cards.)

- Stir-fried vegetables or vegetable side dishes. (Some oriental vegetable dishes are terrific.)

- A taste of rice or noodles. (Generally try to pass on these starches.)

- Your fortune cookie (You can just read the fortune and pass on the starchy cookie.)

- The soups, provided they don't contain MSG.

Poorer choices include:

- Filling up on rice or noodles

- Stir-fried rice—too much starch, too little protein

- Anything with MSG in it

French Restaurants

French cuisine in general offers excellently balanced meals and delicious food. Most often, the meals are made with fresh ingredients and don't contain preservatives and artificial ingredients.

Thinspiration

We love the smaller portions and dining room serenity of French restaurants. Your meals can be pricier than most other kinds of cuisine, but the ambiance is lovely and can be a great teacher. It can show you how to create a calm, beautiful eating experience.

Good choices include:

- Meat, seafood, fish, and poultry entrées

- Vegetables and salads

- Desserts—crème brûlée, mousse, and cheesecake

Poorer choices include:

- Eating too much of that great French bread

- Eating fast without tasting

- Too much French wine

Other Ethnic Cuisines

No matter what the cuisine, whether it's Middle Eastern, German, Russian, South American, Indian, or any other, you can eat in ways that encourage your body to release weight if you follow these guidelines:

- Eat only when you are hungry, at 0.

- Stop eating at or below satisfied, meaning at or below 5.

- Make sure you eat enough high-quality complete protein, at least 15 grams.

- Make sure you get at least one serving of fruit or vegetables and preferably two.

- Avoid eating high-glycemic starches.

Thinspiration

No food is so powerful that it can make you fat. But by eating with wisdom, every food you eat—no matter what type—can support your weight loss and weight maintenance.

The Least You Need to Know

- Eating out is part of life, and you can eat out by ordering regular foods with the confidence that you are getting to your ideal size.

- Eating out does not need to be a reason for weight gain or an inability to lose weight.

- Ordering from the menu is easy when you order what you want and also what offers a healthy balance of protein, carbohydrates, and fats.

- You can dine beautifully without drawing attention to your eating and still reach your ideal size.

- Sharing meals when you eat out and bringing home leftovers make sense for your budget and your size.

- All cuisines are friendly and can support you in getting to your ideal size when you know how to order and eat.

Chapter 27

Special Occasion Eating

In This Chapter

- Eating for the holidays
- Family eating situations
- Celebrating with ease and confidence
- Handling weight-loss comments

Holidays and special occasions can now be enjoyable rather than fattening. No longer do you need to fear the holiday season and packing on 5 to 10 extra pounds. This also means you won't be writing New Year's resolutions to lose weight! You can sail through the holidays—as well as vacations and special occasions such as weddings—with confidence, knowing that you are moving steadily toward your ideal size.

The Tradition of Feasting

Feasting on special occasions has been around about as long as man. Why? Because we like to honor life's rites of passage and religious celebrations, and what better way than to have a party that includes special foods. Feasting days through the ages have included religious holidays, life event celebrations such as marriages and births, season changes, and sporting events, just like today.

Thinspiration

If you have favorite "feast" foods, such as cranberry sauce or rum balls, remember that you can enjoy them at other times of the year as well. This may relieve some of the subtle internal pressure to fill up at the celebration because you won't see that special food again for another year.

In days of old, common folk ate pretty boring and simple foods from day to day. Their meager diet included some meat, some in-season vegetables and fruits, and starches such as bread or rice. It might also include a soupy cereal called gruel … which even sounds boring.

But feast days were different. For instance, the English and American colonists would celebrate by making and eating all sorts of delicacies like plum pudding, mince meat pies, and yes, even fruitcake. (Imagine a bleak, cold winter without any fresh produce. Now take some fruit that was dried or preserved since the summer, add nuts, and bake them into a cake. Fruitcake would have seemed like a delicacy to you, too.) These feast days may have been the only times when the common folk had access to fancy "treat" foods.

The common folk could overindulge at a feast because they seldom, if ever, lived with abundant food in their daily lives. Often, they would struggle to have enough food to get by. At feasts, in a very real sense, they were making up for missed calories. Occasional feasts weren't going to affect their basic body sizes.

Now jump to the present. Do you face food scarcity from day to day? Not likely. You probably enjoy abundance virtually every day. Getting enough calories to fuel your body is as easy as reaching into the pantry or the refrigerator or stopping by a fast-food joint. In fact, finding and obtaining special foods is easy, too. What you can't find at a store within a couple of miles of your house, you can order on the Internet and have delivered directly to your home.

Yet you still want to enjoy special feasts. You still want to make and eat special foods for holidays, weddings, and religious celebrations, even though these treats aren't so special or rare today. The good news is that if you update your perspective about feasts, you can enjoy special foods without overeating them. But to get through feasts with your waistline slim, it takes some thought and planning.

Thanksgiving

Thanksgiving has to be the biggest overeating day in the United States. Our custom is to prepare a turkey with all the trimmings, and the trimmings often includes lots of high-glycemic foods such as mashed potatoes, stuffing, and bread. Plus, our informal custom is to have candy, cheese and crackers, and cookies available all day long. Even just a taste of each of the trimmings can leave a person well above 5 on the hunger scale.

Once we learned to hate the feeling of being really full, we devised a Thanksgiving eating strategy. It's pretty simple:

1. Make sure you are at 0 on the hunger scale before you sit down to dinner. This may mean passing up the appetizers and treats scattered around the house. Save those treats for later or the next day.

2. Only put on your plate modest portions of the foods you like the very best. (Perhaps you prefer dark meat, cranberry sauce, and dressing. Yes, this is an unbalanced meal, but just on this day you can afford it.)

3. Save room for dessert if you like the dessert. In other words, pumpkin pie is great only if you like it.

4. Don't worry about hurting anyone's feelings if you don't eat food they prepared. If the person insists you take some, put the food on your plate, eat one bite, and as you eat, hide the rest under something else!

5. Say a blessing. After all, this is Thanksgiving.

6. Eat slowly and try to make this meal last at least 30 minutes. Many families, when they finally sit down to eat their feast, gulp it down, sometimes in order to not miss the next football game. Bad idea.

7. Eat 0 to 5.

8. Don't go back for seconds unless your hunger number is below 5. The leftovers can be eaten the next day and even the day after that ... and the day after that ... and so on.

9. Have a conversation plan. Perhaps everyone at the table can say what he or she gives thanks for. Make it a fun, upbeat, and bonding time.

Be sure to focus your energy on the purpose of the celebration and the togetherness of family and friends. Let the food be a part of the celebration, not the purpose of the celebration.

Happy Holidays ... Really

You can breeze through the holiday season, that time between Thanksgiving and New Year's Day, and even lose weight or stay at your ideal size. And while you breeze through, you can still enjoy the special foods and treats of the season.

Sound too good to be true? It *is* possible. Other people do it every year. Basically, successful holiday eaters, whether they consciously know it or not, eat from 0 to 5. So can you, but it takes some planning. You are presented with so many opportunities to eat fabulous foods—family parties, office parties, office treats, cocktail parties, open houses, cookie exchanges, and so on. You could go six weeks without ever feeling a simple hunger pang.

Don't be discouraged. Here are some helpful hints to get you through the season smiling:

- Always start eating at 0.

- Go easy on the alcohol. Drinking alcohol can impair your ability to feel your stomach's hunger number.

- Take small tastes of food rather than real portions at parties.

- Make sure you get at least 15 grams of protein at meals. The protein can come in the form of hors d'oeuvres such as shrimp on toothpicks or bacon-wrapped liver.

- You'll be fine if you don't taste or eat everything offered. Really. Party foods are not precious rarities. You'll have other opportunities to eat them.

- Focus on enjoying the people, the conversation, and the ambience. After all, you're at a party.

- Make the party and the people more important than the food.

- If you have multiple parties on the same day, you may want to eat only to a hunger number of 2 or 3 at each party so that you can sample food at each event.

- Always, always stop eating at or below 5 on the hunger scale.

- Maintain your exercise program throughout the holidays.

- Spend time remembering the true meaning of the holidays.

Thinspiration

Since the holidays occur during the dark time of year, when the sun rises late and sets early, some people get the blues from sunlight deprivation. Make sure you get out in the sunshine if you can or use a light box as a source of mood-lifting, full-spectrum light.

Home Alone for the Holidays

Being alone or almost alone for the holidays can be fattening. It's easy to feel left out and sorry for yourself. Maybe you're tempted to console yourself with food. If this is your situation, you can still share the joys of the holidays with others and yourself. Here are a few suggestions:

- Get out and do something for someone else, such as volunteering at a soup kitchen or visiting nursing homes.

- Go to church, mosque, synagogue, or temple and be with other people.

- Take quality time for yourself. Pamper, polish, exercise, read, and catch up with your projects and yourself.

- Eat with wisdom, like you've now learned to do every day. Eat 0 to 5.

- Eat some special holiday treats but carefully and sensuously.

Thinspiration _____

The difference between being alone and being lonely is your state of mind. Do whatever it takes to enjoy yourself and to avoid having a personal pity party.

Parties

Whether you're at a dinner party, a wedding, a Super Bowl celebration, or a neighborhood potluck, apply the same eating principles:

- Make the party, the celebration, and the people more important than the food.

- Start eating at 0 on the hunger scale.

- Be selective about what foods you put on your plate.

- Eat slowly, carefully, and sensuously.

- Save room for dessert or wedding cake if you want some.

- Drink alcohol with caution, remembering that it dulls your hunger sensations, making it tough to know when you've had enough food.

- Stop eating at or below 5.

Thinspiration _____

Learn how to be socially comfortable at parties so that you can have a good time without hiding out near the appetizer tray. If you need to, take a class on small talk or lessons in the art of party going. There really are such classes, and they can be quite helpful.

> CAUTION **Weighty Warning** _____
>
> Because of the nature of potlucks, sometimes you may find very little high-quality protein offered. Just to make sure you get enough protein, maybe you should be the one to bring a protein dish. Foods such as sliced roast or ham, deviled eggs, and a lovely presentation of cheese and fruit make a terrific contribution.

Handling Family and Friends

Why does it seem that people push food on you more when you're on a program to master your weight? Some family events can be emotionally challenging all by themselves; you sure don't need anyone telling you how to eat.

In many families, food is a representation of love. Therefore, a host or hostess may assume his or her love is not being accepted if you don't eat enough food in the person's estimation. Herein lies a big problem. You know that food is not love—at least you should by now—but try explaining that at a family event. It's bound to upset the fun.

The best way to navigate through this minefield at a family gathering is to keep your own counsel. Don't tell anyone that you're on a diet or have lost weight. If anyone mentions it, thank the person for noticing and change the subject. If you're done eating and someone is pushing you to eat more, simply tell the person that you don't have any more room or that you might have some more food later after your food settles. Then you can politely refuse more food later if it's offered.

> CAUTION **Weighty Warning** _____
>
> Be aware that some family members and friends can be uncomfortable with your weight loss and your new way of eating. When you refuse seconds or dessert, they may actually become alarmed. You might be 30 pounds overweight, but they'll claim to be worrying about your health, like you've suddenly become anorexic! Plan now how you'll handle the situation before it happens.

Perhaps your family and friends are seeing you for the first time since you've lost weight. In addition to the compliments, which you will enjoy, you may hear odd comments such as …

"You could stand to put on some weight."

"You're getting too thin."

"Are you sure you aren't getting too thin?"

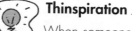

Thinspiration

When someone suggests that you're becoming too thin, thank the person for his or her concern and keep your own counsel. Since you are being successful at losing weight, you can consider it to be a compliment. Your risk of becoming anorexic is miniscule to nonexistent. Only if your body mass index drops below 18 do you need to be concerned.

Such negative comments can wreck your weight-loss program, especially if they come from an authority figure … like Mom or Dad. They can lead you to doubt yourself. You may not even be at your ideal size when you hear such comments. So let's approach this situation logically now because logic can fly out the window when you hear these criticisms.

First, thank the person for his or her concern. Don't explain yourself or make excuses. Instead, change the subject to something about the person questioning you since most people love to talk about themselves. You know you aren't anorexic.

What you don't want to do is start to explain yourself and your eating plan and, in essence, defend yourself. That will make things worse. You and only you know if you are on track and how hard you have worked to get to the size you've attained. Remember, in their own way, the people who ask these kinds of questions are naysayers even if they're family and friends. When it comes to weight, you're much more likely to get bad advice than good advice from others.

The Least You Need to Know

- Feasting for special occasions is an age-old human custom.
- We live in an age of abundance in which special foods formerly reserved for feasts are widely available every day at food stores and over the Internet.
- At special events, focus on the celebration and not the food.
- Overeating during the holidays and at parties is not a requirement; in fact, you should plan to continue to lose weight and enjoy the parties.
- Be prepared to handle comments from family and friends about your new weight and new ways of eating.

Chapter 28

The Support You Need

In This Chapter

- Finding the right support group
- Creating your own group
- Celebrating wins
- Supporting yourself

People who lose weight in groups tend to lose more weight and maintain their new sizes more easily. The mutual support and encouragement helps you tackle the challenges and keeps you going through the ups and downs of reaching your ideal size.

Needing support is normal. By nature, on our journeys through life, we seek companionship and soul mates. Your journey to reach your ideal size is no different. A personal support group will be a huge help. Its members are your cheerleaders, a sounding board, and a place to discuss your eating concerns. Whether your support group is just one other person or 20, being part of a group can make a difference in your success. The good news is that going the distance alone isn't necessary.

Support Helps

As you know already from experience, losing weight presents many potential road-blocks and some difficult terrain. We're referring to such things as late-night eating binges or unconsciously polishing off the whole bucket of popcorn at the movie. Perhaps in a nervous social setting you might chomp down on dozens of appetizers or experience emotional upheaval that leads you to drown your sorrows in a quart of ice cream!

Then there's the question of how to emotionally deal with the slip-ups, the little binges, the eating past 5 on the hunger scale. Picking yourself back up and rebuilding your weight-loss resolve can be challenging. Some days it can seem easier to just give up and forget about trying to get to your ideal size.

You don't have to do it alone. Let's repeat that: You don't have to do it alone. A support group can give you the encouragement to keep on keeping on—one day at a time or one phone call at a time until you reach your ideal size.

Support groups come in many varieties. Here are some of your choices:

♦ **Formal commercially sponsored groups.** These are usually part of national weight-loss programs such as Weight Watchers. Meetings cost about $10 per session and are based on the eating philosophy of the sponsor. But beware. You may have to step on the scale or do other unproductive activities, so preview the group before you join. If you don't feel positively motivated after your first meeting, don't go back.

Thinspiration

If a weight-loss support group fits you, join and stay with it. If it doesn't fit, find another option. A support group that doesn't fit is like a shoe that's too small. No matter what you do, it still isn't going to fit. You don't need to bend and conform so that you can fit into the weight-loss group.

♦ **Internet support from such sites as eDiets and iVillage.** Since the Internet is perpetually available, you can sign on at any time for information and encouragement. Many of these sites have ongoing chat rooms. Some offer online consultations with registered dietitians and psychologists. (Lucy's website at www.LucyBeale. com and Sandy's website at www. NutritionSandy.com offer information and e-mail support.)

♦ **Ongoing groups in your town.** These are often listed on community bulletin boards and in the local newspapers. Sometimes attendance is free, sometimes not.

♦ **A group sponsored by a weight-loss coach or registered dietitian or by your church.** Most likely there's a fee for these groups, but it can be money well spent.

♦ **Your own support group.** You can form your own small group of friends or acquaintances that meets together for lunch, dinner, at each other's homes, or virtually via the Internet. You'll learn more about this in the next section.

Thinspiration

Professional weight-loss coaches and nutritionists sometimes hold group classes over a period of time. These may be held in offices, health clubs, and recreation centers. I, Lucy, hold conference-call phone classes on a weekly basis to let individuals participate from anywhere in the United States. (I've even done classes with callers from Canada, Australia, and the United Kingdom! You can enroll for the classes at www.LucyBeale.com.)

Make sure you're comfortable with the emphasis of the professional coach. Some have a tendency to become focused on only one aspect of weight control. For instance, some focus almost exclusively on counting calories or fat grams. Others are little more than exercise-aholics. You want someone who takes a whole body—and whole mind—approach that's informative, upbeat, and inspiring.

Make sure the support group you choose is uplifting and positive. In some groups, people become very emotional and delve into their heavy-duty life conditions and challenges. Decide if that feels good to you and, most of all, if it ultimately supports you in getting to your ideal size. Don't get hooked into a group that's little more than a "gripe-whine" session.

In addition, when choosing a support group, be sure to attend about three sessions to find out how it feels and if it meets your needs. Use the following criteria for your decision:

♦ Are the people in the group dealing with many of the same eating and weight issues that you are?

♦ Do the people in the group have about the same amount of weight to lose as you do?

♦ Are the group members losing weight or just talking about it?

♦ Is the flow of the conversation uplifting and positive?

♦ Do the group members really want to get to their ideal size, and are they willing to do what it takes?

- Are you comfortable with the weight-loss and eating philosophies presented?

- Are the members celebrating their wins at each meeting and getting positive acknowledgement and reinforcement for their progress?

If the group feels right, join it and be an active participant so that you get value and make progress toward your goals. If the time comes when you need to move on, do so. It's perfectly fine to leave the group when it no longer meets your needs. Don't ever let yourself be shamed into staying by the group leader or by the other members.

Create Your Support Group

Putting together and orchestrating a support group is an excellent way for you to reach your goals, especially if you're willing to remain the group leader. When you devote the time and energy to help the group succeed, you'll accelerate reaching your ideal size and staying there.

First, determine what you want for your group in terms of time, cost, number of people, forms of interaction, and eating and weight philosophy. Since you already know plenty of people who also want to get to their ideal size, let them know you want to start a group. Set up the format and guidelines and get started.

Here are suggestions for format:

- **Weekly meetings in person.** To succeed, group members must really commit to get to the meetings. The advantage is that you support each other's weight-loss efforts from week to week, and you'll literally see how others are doing. That in itself can be motivating. If weekly face-to-face meetings are inconvenient or take too much time, use the phone as mentioned below.

Thinspiration

Consider starting a weight-loss support group if the groups that are already available don't meet your needs. It can be fun, strengthen friendships, and add a new dimension to your life. But mostly, you should expect the group to help you and everyone in the group reach your ideal size.

- **Weekly meetings on the phone.** Conference call or set up a daisy chain using three-way calling. These meetings are easy to get to—they're as close as your phone—and can be done from virtually anywhere. It's a good idea for your group to get together in person every month or at least every other month.

- **Live online chat.** Your group can schedule to "meet" via the Internet at the same time. Generally speaking, if you're willing to schedule an e-mail chat, you might as well schedule a phone meeting, but an Internet group meeting might meet some groups' needs.

◆ **Frequent e-mail contact.** This is excellent for between-meeting contact and follow-up. If you add a threaded-discussion format, you can follow and discuss topics over time.

◆ **One-on-one phone calls for emergencies.** The group members can exchange telephone numbers and agree to call each other for support. The support call helps soothe the feelings of isolation and fear that occur when a person is highly stressed, overeats, and even when he or she wants to binge.

In support groups, people come and go, so be prepared to accept the flow and continue to invite others to join your group. People who are losing weight tend to be skittish about such things as accountability, progress, and bumps along the way. Some will drop out. Keep the group upbeat about losing and adding members.

The Group Agenda

Keep the meetings flowing and fun. In about one hour, people can get support, develop camaraderie, and leave feeling motivated.

Here's a suggested agenda:

◆ Open with an inspirational quote or saying.

◆ Celebrate wins. Have each person share his or her wins for the week. If this takes too long, have each person write down their 10 wins for the week, pair up, and share in pairs. Acknowledge each other for the wins. It doesn't matter how big or small the win; what matters is that wins are acknowledged. Ooh and aah about everyone's wins and successes. Applaud. We all need this.

◆ Address problems and solutions. Give each person the opportunity to present any roadblocks encountered during the past week. The group can brainstorm solutions. This way, everyone in the group learns to think creatively about eating and emotional situations, and they learn how to change their behavior and attitudes. The group members learn how to prepare for challenges they may face as they master their eating and their weight.

Thinspiration

Support groups are effective when the members are getting results and when they are finding solutions to their eating problems. Plus, seeing group members lose weight motivates others to do the same, as in "If she can do it, so can I." Keep your meetings fun and productive.

As with other important parts of your life, writing down your weekly weight-loss action plan will help you get it done. There's something about committing plans to paper that gives the tasks more focus and boosts your determination. Your written plan can include your goals, the key steps you're planning to follow, and some way to mark off or record your wins.

- ◆ Introduce educational items. Each week a different person can present new information about nutrition, exercise, or research on weight loss. Occasionally invite a guest speaker such as an exercise expert or nutritionist.

- ◆ Commit for the upcoming week. Each person makes a personal commitment to his or her action plan for the next week. The weekly action plan includes exercise, eating, affirmations, and general goal setting.

- ◆ Offer a thought for the week. Make it an inspirational or fun moment.

Consider sharing the responsibility for managing the group and meetings with several other people. That way, those who share group leadership become more committed to everyone's success, which in turn will motivate them toward personal success as well.

Going It Alone

If groups don't fit for you, create your own personal support system. You can even hold your own meeting with yourself. At a minimum, once a week take the time to assess your progress. You can even follow the preceding agenda.

Thinspiration

Celebrating weight-loss wins sets you up for more and more success. Review your day and your week in terms of what you accomplished, not based on what you left undone or the mistakes made. View your journey to your ideal size from the perspective of the hero's path. The mere undertaking of mastering your weight and your eating makes you a hero or heroine.

Make sure you celebrate your wins. A win can be a big thing, such as fitting into a smaller pair of jeans, or it can be something small. An example of a win is not overeating when you go out to dinner or passing up the donuts at the office because you weren't at 0 on the hunger scale. Write your wins down either daily or weekly so that you have written proof of your progress. All wins are significant. They represent the steps you've taken toward reaching your ideal size.

At your personal progress meeting with yourself, work out your weekly action plan. Schedule your exercise sessions for the next week. You might even make a grocery list to stock up on the foods you most enjoy that fit your nutrition plan. Look ahead to any parties and celebrations and plan your approach. For example, plan how to arrive already at 0, what to wear, and how to have the most enjoyable time.

Finally, keep your motivation strong by using positive self-talk and by finding quotes or information on how to keep your resolve and commitment strong. You might even reread chapters in this book that will reinvigorate your determination.

The Least You Need to Know

- ◆ People in weight-loss support groups tend to lose more weight and more easily stay at their ideal size.

- ◆ Whether you join a commercial support group, a group in your community, or an online version, check it out first to make sure it works for you and meets your needs.

- ◆ A good alternative is to set up your own support group with friends or colleagues.

- ◆ You can hold your own support meeting with yourself to support your progress and stay on track toward attaining your ideal size.

Chapter **29**

Maintaining Your Ideal Size

In This Chapter

- ◆ Solidifying your success
- ◆ Your good-bye fat self letter
- ◆ Moving beyond your weight issue
- ◆ What to do if you gain a few pounds
- ◆ Dressing at your ideal size

Maintaining your weight loss involves many, many aspects of your life. Certainly what and how you eat make a big difference in staying at your ideal size, but how you think and how you live are also important.

You want to be truly finished with being overweight. Permanently. Forever. You don't want any part of your former overweight self hanging around as you live the rest of your life. You want the "new you" to be "the real you" for the rest of your life.

Sometimes formerly overweight individuals constantly fret about food and dieting. They can't seem to let go of the issue. We don't want that to happen with you. When your weight loss is complete, when you reach your ideal size, it's time (with a capital T) for you to bid a fond farewell to your fat self and get on with other, more interesting aspects of life.

The Good-bye Fat Self Letter

Write a good-bye letter to your fat self. To sign and seal the deal, write a good old-fashioned "Dear John" letter. Declare to your fat self that the relationship is over—*finis!*—and you're starting a new life with your thin self.

Are you ready? Then let's do it. Set aside 15 minutes to a half-hour and, using pen and paper, write your letter. Tell your fat self that you appreciate all it has done for you. Thank it for all of the lessons it presented to you. Acknowledge all the lessons learned along the way.

Thinspiration

Try writing a good-bye fat self letter even before you have reached your ideal size. You may be surprised at how hard it is to really say good-bye, but doing so early on can help you align your mindset with your goals.

Tell your fat self that you won't be needing it any longer for protection and padding, that you have found other ways to meet those needs. Then say a fond good-bye and let your fat self go.

Read the letter aloud and, if you want, create a ceremony (such as lighting a candle) to say your formal good-byes. Then release your fat self forever and welcome in your new ideal size.

Your good-bye letter to your fat self should be as personal as possible, but we're including a brief sample to help you get started.

Dear fat self,

You're going to find this hard to believe, but it's finally time for us to part ways. Forever. We've been together for ___ years, through good times and bad, through thick and, well, not exactly thin. But the relationship is over. I don't plan to be overweight ever again. You taught me a lot about life and about myself. Now I know how to eat and live without you.

You brought me lots of pain, too. Because of you, I've been unhappy. I've been through more clothes sizes than I care to think about. You've made shopping unpleasant. You've made food seem like some evil that I couldn't resist. You've made me cry. You've even made my health worse. I'm tired of it. It's over. I will not—repeat, NOT—be a fat person ever again. I'm much happier at my ideal size. I look better, feel better, and know I'm healthier. I plan to ignore that I ever knew you. So, adios. Sayonara. Auf wiedersehen. Good-bye!

Your good-bye letter can cover very specific issues to which you want to say "good-bye." You can itemize the pains you've personally experienced and the past frustrations you've had trying to lose weight. To further solidify letting go of your previous fat self, we recommend that you use the exercise in the next section.

Thinspiration

What do you do if you're stuck at a certain size and your weight just won't budge? Write a good-bye letter to that size. In the letter, ask to be given all the lessons from your current size so that you can move on to the next size. We've seen people lose a size within days of writing this letter.

Moving Beyond

Letting go of your fatter self should be easy, shouldn't it? Not necessarily. Even though you didn't like being overweight, it was familiar to you. The truth is, you and your overweight self spent lots of time together. You were, after all, on an intimate first-name basis.

This exercise lets you finally cut the ties that bind you to that old persona. Using the exercise, you'll complete a quick makeover that will put you emotionally, mentally, and spiritually in sync with your ideal size.

The "Moving Beyond" Exercise Steps

Here's how it works. Give yourself a half-hour or more and, with notepad and pen in hand, do the following:

- ◆ On the top of the first page write, "Why I am thankful for having had a weight issue." List what you learned and whatever else comes to mind. List items such as protection, padding, and avoidance of hard choices.

- ◆ On the next page write, "What I leave behind with my weight issue." Save space to list any personality qualities you want to leave behind, along with activities, big-size clothing, relationships, and so on. Be sure to add overeating to the list as well as telling yourself that you're fat.

- ◆ On the third page write, "Who I forgive and why." Be sure to include yourself. List people you know as well as media figures and magazines that have made you feel bad or have affected your eating behavior. You can even forgive fast-food restaurants for introducing the "supersize" meal!

<table>
<tr><td>

Body of Knowledge

In addition to helping you move beyond your weight issue, the "moving beyond" exercise will also work for other aspects of your life. You can use similar questions for changing jobs, changing relationships, selling your home, and even to finalize the grieving process. We've seen people work small miracles of healing in their lives by using this simple and elegant exercise.

</td></tr>
</table>

◆ On the fourth page write, "What I learned from having a weight issue." Some of your answers could be duplicates from the preceding lists, but keep on writing everything that comes to mind. For instance, you've now learned how to eat as a thin person, how to master your weight, and how to take good care of yourself.

◆ On the fifth page write, "What I look forward to as I live at my ideal size." List your dreams, clothing, health, fitness level, activities, relationships, and career.

Take your time and fill out each page, listing your answers to the questions. Just write what comes to mind. It may take a while, so don't feel rushed. Then set an appointment with yourself for your "moving beyond" ceremony.

The "Moving Beyond" Ceremony

At your "moving beyond" ceremony, you can light candles, burn incense, go to a beautiful location, or do whatever pleases you. Then read your lists aloud and enjoy the feeling of release from your weight issue once and for all. Yes, you can even burn the pages at the end if that will add to your sense of completion.

Thinspiration

Part of your ceremony can include giving away overweight clothes to the thrift shop and paring down your wardrobe to fit your ideal size. Resolve never to need fat clothes again.

The ceremony isn't just for show. Our clients who take the time to do the "moving beyond" exercise and ceremony are much more successful at staying at their ideal size. It empowers them to walk away with finality from any attachment they have to their former weightier selves. It solidifies their weight loss and their commitment to a new lighter self.

If Those Jeans Get Tight

If you ever find your jeans getting tight, you must take immediate action. We can't emphasize this enough. Don't procrastinate. Don't get depressed or anxious. Take action. It is a whole lot easier to lose 3 or 4 pounds than to lose 20. By taking immediate action, you should be able to fit into those jeans within 5 to 10 days, maybe by the next weekend!

Gaining a couple of pounds happens to most people from time to time whether or not they were ever overweight. Short-term gain comes from overeating and also with age and stress.

Here's what to do when your clothes feel tight:

1. Start keeping a food diary that lists your beginning and ending hunger numbers. Record everything you put in your mouth except water.

2. Only eat when your stomach hunger number is 0 and stop eating when you're satisfied and before you're full—that is, stop at or below 5.

3. Make sure you're getting a good balance of high-quality protein, fruits, and vegetables. (We also recommend consuming about two tablespoons of essential fatty acids daily.)

4. Keep up your exercise program. If you have stopped exercising, start again immediately and work up wisely to your former intensity levels of cardio, strength training, and stretching.

5. Cut out or cut back on high-glycemic foods, namely the starches, and get most of your carbohydrates from fruits and vegetables.

6. Start writing your affirmations again every day. Write, "I, (*fill in your name*), am now a naturally healthy and thin person. I wear a size (*insert ideal size*), and I do what thin people do." Write this in your notebook 10 times daily.

7. Use the stress reducers listed in Chapter 8 as a way to reduce stress and stop emotional eating.

8. Review other information in this book and make note of where you may have gotten off track. Then take positive action to correct your situation.

If you do the preceding, you can expect quick results. Your body at its ideal size has established a new set point, and it wants to stay there. So help it out. It will respond.

Dressing at Your Ideal Size

You're at your ideal size. At last you can wear all those fashionable clothes you've longed to wear. Perhaps you've noticed that people who are at their ideal size often wear different styles of clothing than people who are overweight. You have many more choices now that you've reached your ideal size. You'll never need to wear vertical stripes just because they make you look thinner—you are thinner!

We suggest that you reinforce your commitment to yourself by avoiding "overweight" types of clothes. Take a look at the following lists, and you'll get a sense of the clothing that will show off your new body.

In general, give up wearing these "overweight" clothing styles:

- ◆ Big and long over-blouses and tunics
- ◆ Elastic-stretch waistbands
- ◆ Stretch pants designed to accommodate weight gain
- ◆ Big, flowing dresses and slacks
- ◆ Tent-shaped dresses
- ◆ Big, loose, long, and flowing jackets or coats
- ◆ Clothing purchased in "big people" shops
- ◆ Huge sweatshirts

Instead, you might choose:

- ◆ Belted slacks
- ◆ Tailored slacks and pantsuits
- ◆ Form-fitting stretch jeans
- ◆ T-shirts and torso-hugging knits
- ◆ Tailored blazers and jackets
- ◆ Shorter skirts when they're in style (and even when they aren't!)
- ◆ Sexy heels and sandals
- ◆ Sundresses and evening wear that show some skin

> **Body of Knowledge**
>
> If dressing as a thin person is new to you, enlist the help of a professional wardrobe coach or a knowledgeable salesperson. This type of person can help you coordinate your wardrobe so that your clothes meet your new lifestyle needs and you don't overspend your budget.

Choose clothing that tastefully and lovingly reveals rather than hides your body. You have done a lot of work to master your weight. It's perfectly fine to show off your success.

The Need for Compassion

You know firsthand the pain and sadness of being overweight. You also know the prejudice and ridicule you endured when you were bigger. So make a firm commitment to never look down on or criticize others who have yet to reach their ideal size. You owe it to yourself and, in a sense, to the world.

No one should have to feel the pain of low self-esteem and prejudiced treatment because of his or her weight. Now that you've mastered your weight, you can be part of the solution, not part of the problem. Here are some suggestions for how to help others:

Thinspiration

Give the gifts of understanding and compassion to others who are still struggling with their weight issue. Follow the golden rule. Treat others just as you wish you had been treated when you were overweight.

- Respect the challenges that others still face.

- Never become preachy about losing weight.

- Graciously accept compliments without gloating.

- Offer advice only when asked for it.

- When asked, let people know that they can master their weight.

Because you've mastered getting to your ideal size, you've demonstrated that the epidemic of obesity and being overweight can be solved—one person at a time. You've actually helped make the world a healthier place. If others ask how you mastered your weight issue, by all means share your success story so that you can help them experience the joy and freedom you now have. But be sure to do so graciously and kindly.

The Least You Need to Know

- Writing a good-bye letter to your fat self lets you solidify your weight-loss success.

- Use the "moving beyond" exercise to once and for all walk away from your weight issue.

- Should your jeans get tight, immediately get back on track by recording your food intake, eating 0 to 5, and using affirmations.

- Dress as a thin person to enhance your body; do not hide it.

- Direct the compassion and forgiveness you have developed toward yourself and your weight issue to others who are still struggling with their weight.

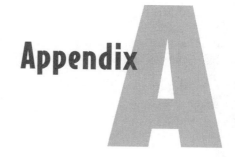

Glossary

adrenal glands   Two glands located in the stomach that produce hormones related to stress, including adrenaline and cortisol.

adrenaline   A hormone produced in response to stress that directly affects the brain as a stimulus. It is known as the fight-or-flight hormone.

affirmation   A positive statement declaring that you already have what you want.

amino acid   The basic unit that makes up protein. There are essential amino acids that we must get from our food to maintain health. Nonessential amino acids can be synthesized in the body but are also required for health.

appetite   A natural biological desire for food that may vary daily.

autonomic nervous system   The part of the nervous system that controls involuntary responses in the body.

basal metabolism rate (BMR)   The number of calories your body needs for basic involuntary processes such as breathing, eyes blinking, heart beating, digesting, and so on.

bitter orange   An herb used in some diet supplements that has mild amphetamine-like stimulants.

body mass index (BMI)   A measure of the relationship between height and weight.

calorie   A measurement of the energy contained in food when digested and assimilated by the body.

cardio/aerobic   Cardiovascular exercise that strengthens the heart, builds lung oxygen capacity, and releases endorphins. It needs to be sustained for a minimum of 20 minutes.

cholesterol   A waxy, fat-like substance. Dietary cholesterol is found in foods of animal origin. Blood cholesterol is manufactured by the liver and found in every body cell. Cholesterol is needed for many functions of a healthy body.

complementary proteins   Two or more incomplete proteins that together contain all the essential amino acids to equal a complete protein.

complete proteins   Foods that contain all of the essential amino acids.

constipation   The irregular, difficult, or sluggish passage of stool.

cortisol   A hormone manufactured by the adrenal glands in response to stress. It facilitates fat storage and affects the immune system.

country mallow   Another name used for ephedra or ma huang, the herb that is often used in thermogenic weight loss supplements that has amphetamine-type stimulants and may have harmful side effects.

eating 0 to 5   Eating when you are hungry and stopping when you are satisfied, before you are full. Do this by using the hunger scale to rate the hunger and fullness of your stomach. Zero means that your stomach has hunger pangs and is empty. Five means that you have had enough food but not too much food. Seven means that you are full, and 10 means that you are stuffed.

eating beautifully   Eating in an environment that is peaceful, health giving, and fun.

effective weight-loss system   A system that incorporates behavior, nutrition, and exercise along with education to help a person maintain his or her ideal size.

endorphins   Chemical agents released by the body that stimulate the brain to feel good, released during vigorous exercise.

energy   The fuel required by the body to power body processes. Energy is obtained from carbohydrate, protein, fat, and alcohol.

enzyme   A protein that facilitates chemical reactions in the body.

ephedra   An herb, also known as ma huang and country mallow, used in many diet supplements that has amphetamine-type stimulants and that may have harmful side effects.

essential amino acids These cannot be made by the body. They must come from food sources.

essential fatty acids Dietary fats that the body requires for health.

fasting The act of abstaining from eating food for a period of time, usually one or more days.

fiber That portion of a plant that the human body cannot digest. It provides indigestible bulk, which encourages the normal elimination of body wastes.

food combining Eating more than one kind of carbohydrate that contains incomplete proteins so that, when combined, you are consuming all the essential amino acids found in complete proteins such as meat and eggs. For instance, eating beans and rice together will provide you with all the essential amino acids. You don't have to eat the combined foods at the same meal as long as you eat them within the same 24-hour period.

forgiveness The act of pardoning others or yourself without harboring resentment.

free radicals Unstable, hyperactive molecules that move around in the body, damaging healthy cells and tissues.

glycemic index A measure of a carbohydrate's ability to raise the body's blood sugar.

good nutrition The state that exists when the body has been receiving the required amounts of the nutrients it needs to function properly.

gym A health club, athletic center, recreation center, or other location that offers exercise facilities.

high-glycemic Rapidly digested carbohydrates, usually starches, that cause a quick rise in blood sugar and insulin levels which can lead to increased fat storage.

hormone A chemical substance produced by body organs that alters the functional activity of various organs in the body.

hunger A physical sensation triggered by hormones and blood chemistry that tells you your body needs fuel.

hunger scale A numeric system designed to help you rate the fullness of your stomach. See *eating 0 to 5*.

ideal size The size that keeps you healthy and makes you happy.

incomplete proteins Foods containing some but not all of the essential amino acids.

inertia   This law of physics states that a body in motion tends to stay in motion and a body at rest tends to stay at rest. This law applies to exercise programs and body movement in general.

insulin   A hormone secreted by the pancreas in response to rising blood sugar.

intention   A statement that is the subset of a primary affirmation.

ketosis   A body condition that occurs when the body burns fat without enough glucose.

light box   An electrical lighting device that provides natural, full-spectrum light.

liposuction   A surgical procedure in which body fat is suctioned from various fat storage areas of the body.

long-cooking oatmeal   Steel-cut oats, usually imported from Ireland. Available at health food and food specialty stores.

ma huang   Another name for the herb ephedra that is used in thermogenic weight-loss supplements that has amphetamine-type stimulants and may have harmful side effects.

macronutrients   Nutrients required in relatively large amounts, such as calcium and phosphorus.

metabolism   The sum total of all chemical reactions that take place in living cells. Also, the rate at which a person burns calories.

micronutrients   Nutrients required in relatively small amounts, such as vanadium, which is beneficial for thyroid metabolism and boron, which is important to bone health.

mineral   An inorganic compound occurring in nature and required by the body for normal metabolic functioning.

neurotransmitter   A chemical produced by brain cells (neurons) that increases or decreases brain activity.

nonessential amino acids   These are amino acids that can be synthesized in the body from the essential amino acids and are required for health.

nutrients   The chemical components of food that the body requires to perform the various activities associated with living.

nutrition   The relationship of food to the well-being of the body.

obesity   An excess of body fat. Guidelines: 30 percent or more over the suggested weight for height or having a BMI of 30 or higher.

overweight   An excess amount of body weight, including fat, muscle, bone, and water. Guidelines: Women having over 25 percent body fat, men over 20 percent; women having a waist size over 35 inches with a high BMI; men having a waist size over 40 inches with a high BMI; anyone with a BMI of 25 to 29.9.

oxidation   The process by which the tissues of the body make the energy in food available to the body.

parasympathetic nervous system   The part of the autonomic nervous system that calms the brain and body.

pedometer   A small device that counts each step taken. It is usually worn on a belt or belt loop.

phytonutrients   The chemicals in plants that protect them from harsh environmental conditions and that give them color, flavor, and aroma. These are known to aid the body in promoting immune function and preventing diseases such as cancer and heart disease.

Pilates   A total-body conditioning approach that emphasizes both stretching and strength-training, developed by Joseph Pilates. Also known as core conditioning.

plateau   No evidence of weight loss, inches lost, or decrease in body fat for four weeks or more.

recommended dietary allowance (RDA)   In the United States, the level of dietary intake of essential nutrients considered to be sufficient to meet the nutritional needs of most healthy individuals based on age, sex, body size, activity, and diet.

registered dietitian   A nutrition professional qualified through education and mandatory recognized professional affiliation to participate, advise, and direct in the field of nutrition.

satiety   A mechanism to tell the body that it has had enough food.

saturated fat   Fats found in most animal foods and some plants. Saturated fat is solid at room temperature.

scale   A machine that measures a person's specific gravity in relation to the earth. This measurement is called a person's weight.

scorecard   A personal exercise progress and activity record.

semolina   A hard durum wheat that's high in gluten and is used commercially in many pasta products.

serotonin   A neurotransmitter in the brain that lifts mood.

spinning A group exercise activity offered at health clubs that uses stationary bikes. The instructor sets the pace to promote a sustained high-level cardio workout.

starvation metabolism The slowing of the basal metabolic rate, causing the body to burn calories slower and build up fat stores.

strength training A program of exercises that uses resistance to stress the muscles so that they get stronger.

stress soothers Positive, inspiring, and uplifting alternatives to eating for stress release.

sympathetic nervous system The part of the autonomic nervous system that moves the body into fight-or-flight mode.

synthesize The process of manufacturing a complex substance from a simpler substance.

Tibetans Five simple exercises that are performed 21 times each. They promote health and aid in balancing hormonal activity. When done daily, they help eliminate double chins and middle age spread.

trans-fatty acids A type of saturated fat formed during a manufacturing process called hydrogenation, which makes the fat more shelf stable and solid at room temperature. Current research shows that these fats cause a rise in blood cholesterol levels and are the unhealthiest types of fat.

tryptophan An amino acid that is converted to serotonin in the brain.

unsaturated fat Fat that is liquid at room temperature. It is found naturally in most plant oils and some animal foods.

vitamin An organic substance required by the body in trace amounts for normal metabolic functioning.

weight-loss program A combination of an organized eating plan, an exercise program, and behavior modifications to assist in getting to and maintaining your ideal size.

yoga Stretching-oriented exercise that promotes balance, strength, and flexibility. It originated in India thousands of years ago.

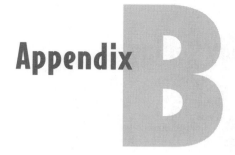

Appendix B

Resources

Here's where to find the products we mention as beneficial for your weight loss and exercise success. In addition, we have given you a list of our favorite exercise videos and included the weight loss books we discussed.

Back Roller, Also Called Ma Roller

Body Tools
www.bodytools.com
1-800-845-6202
Fax: 415-382-8897

Be Thin in Body, Mind & Spirit CDs and Audiotapes

www.LucyBeale.com
1-888-443-1979 (during business hours)
24-hour fax line: 480-443-3522

Body Rolling

Body Rolling
book, video, and balls
www.bodylogic.com

FitBall Body Therapy
book, video, and balls
www.fitball.com

Clickers and Pedometers

Available at sporting goods stores.

Exercise Videos

www.collagevideo.com—This site has a terrific selection of tapes for Pilates, yoga, cardio, fitness ball, and more. Here you can find these instructors and videos that we recommend:

- ◆ Jennifer Kries' Pilates Method: The Method Precision Toning, 3-D Toning, Precision Pilates, and The Perfect Mix. Jennifer mixes Pilates with dance, yoga, and weight training. She explains each exercise clearly and we like her warmth and style.

- ◆ FitBall Lower-Body Challenge and Upper Body Challenge. The moves on these two videos are terrific for toning, but the video is challenging. If you are just starting out, go slow, don't get intimidated, and work up carefully to full speed.

- ◆ Moira Stott: Pilates New Matwork Series, Flexband Workout, Fitness Circle Workout, Power Circle Workout. Moira is a revered world expert in Pilates. Her deep understanding of body movement comes through in her videos.

www.FitBall.com—This site has Colleen Craig's On The Ball video which offers great instruction on Pilates for beginning FitBall users.

www.stottpilates.com—This site offers all of Moira Stott's videos plus videos for using the Reformer equipment. Choose from Essential Reformer, Intermediate Reformer, Advanced Reformer I and II, and Power Reformer videos.

Fitness Ball

www.fitball.com

1-800-752-2255

Fitness Circle

www.pilates-studio.com

www.stottpilates.com

Glycemic Index

www.mendosa.com/gi.htm

Internet Weight-Loss Sites

www.eDiets.com

www.CyberDiets.com

www.iVillage.com

www.nutrition.about.com

Light Box

Happy Lite
cost is $229
www.gaiam.com

Naturally Healthy & Thin E-mail Newsletter

www.LucyBeale.com (to sign up)

Pilates Reformer Equipment

www.pilates-studio.com

www.QVC.com

(This equipment works well for home use and costs about $500; the Reformer folds up and rolls away for storage.)

Protein Counter

The Protein Counter, by Annette B. Natow, Pocket Books, March 1997.
You can also print it from the website at www.aakp.org/calorieerg.htm.

Rebounding Boots

www.HealthMattersNow.net

1-888-333-2078

Supplements

All of these, unless otherwise noted, are widely available at health food stores.

- ◆ Electrolytes:
  Emergen-C comes in individual packets and mixes instantly with water (many different flavors).
  Knudsen's Recharge Drink is bottled fruit juice with electrolytes.

- ◆ Essential amino acids: There are dozens of good amino acid supplements at health food stores. We suggest you try several and see which brand works best for you.

- ◆ Digestive enzymes: NOW Super Enzyme Caps

- ◆ Essential fatty acids (EFAs):
  Dr. Udo Oil
  The Total EFA

- ◆ Greens drinks: Greens Plus—www.greensplus.com

- ◆ Liquid B vitamins: B Total Sublingual

- ◆ Necessary sugars: Ambrotose from Mannatech at www.mannatech.com or 1-800-281-4469

- ◆ Trace minerals: ConcenTrace Trace Mineral Tablets

Tibetan Exercise Books

Ancient Secret of the Fountain of Youth, Book 1. Peter Kelder, Bernie S. Siegel, Doubleday, February 1998.
This is the original book, reprinted from the 1939 edition.

Ancient Secret of the Fountain of Youth, Book 2. Peter Kelder, Bernie S. Siegel, Doubleday, February 1999.
This updated and expanded book explains why the exercises are so effective and includes beginner exercises for building up strength for doing the complete set of five exercises.

Weighted Shoes for Walking

866-397-2639

www.5pillars.com/4health

Weight Loss Books

The Carbohydrate Addicts Diet, Rachael F. Heller, Ph.D., Richard Heller, Ph.D., E. P. Dalton, March 1993.

Dr. Atkins New Diet Revolution, Robert C. Atkins M.D., Avon, December 2001.

Protein Power, Michael R. Eades and Mary Dan Eades, Bantam, December 1997.

Sugar Busters, H. Leighton Steward; Sam S. Andrews, M.D.; Morrison C. Bethea, M.D.; Luis A. Balart, M.D., Ballantine, May 1998.

The Zone, Barry Sears, Ph.D, with Bill Lawren, Harper Collins, June 1995.

Yoga

Bikram's Beginning Yoga Class, Bikram Choudhury, J.P. Tarcher, August 2000.

Index

F

designing a food plan, 158
modern-day, 231-232
videotapes, cardio/aerobic,
185
visualizations, 47
vital nutrients, 120
vitamins, 142-143
B vitamins, 144

W

waist/hip ratio, 39
walking, 185
warmth, as stress soother, 84
water, 140-141
as stress soother, 90
getting in water to reduce
stress, 84
purified water, 142
weather, as barrier to exercising, 204
web-based eating plans, 225
e-miracles, 226
recommended programs,
226
weight training
free weights, 187
weight-training machines,
188
Weight Watchers, 220-222
weight-burning foods, 238
weight-loss plans, 209
alternative choices, 249
bedtime formulations,
252
body wraps, 252-253
herbal supplements,
250-251
hypnosis, 253-254
miraculous weight loss
products, 254
one-on-one coaching,
253

blood-type diet, 234
common-sense food sug-
gestions, 215
accessibility of foods,
217
avoiding processed
starches, 217
balance, 215
liquid diet warnings,
216
meeting fat needs, 216
meeting fruit and veg-
etable requirements,
216
cost, 214
fasting, 230-231
food combining, 234
frequent-eater plans, 236
high-protein diets,
237-238
lifestyle criteria, 210
fit with current lifestyle,
212
lifetime approach, 211
simplicity, 211-212
low-fat diets, 239
maintenance plans, 217
Monday madness, 210
no-sugar diets, 241
Paleo diet, 235-236
prepackaged food diets,
241-242
specialty diet systems, 242
vegetarianism, 231-233
weight-burning foods, 238
working your biology, 212
health promotion, 214
overeating, 213
safety checks, 213-214
starvation, 213
zone eating, 240-241
weight-loss programs, 219
evaluating, 223-224
Jenny Craig, 222
Overeaters Anonymous,
225

prepackaged foods, 220
web-based eating plans,
225
e-miracles, 226
recommended pro-
grams, 226
Weight Watchers, 220-222
weight-training machines,
188
Wellbutrin, 246

X-Y-Z

Xenical, 245
xylose, 115

yeast overgrowth, 146
yo-yo dieting syndrome, 68
yoga, 89, 188

zone eating, 240-241

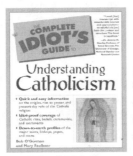
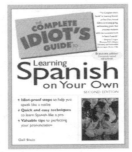
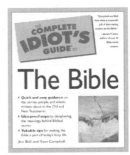
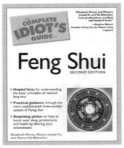
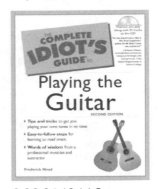
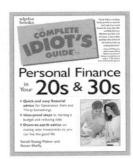
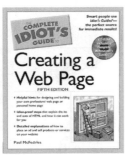
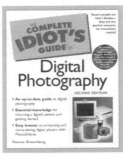
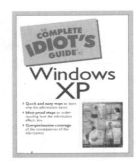